CONTENTS

ACKNOWLEDGEMENTS

Thanks to the friends who have been involved with this project and those who supported me during the nights hunched over the computer.

JST

To the usual suspects – you know who you are. Thanks for all the support in this third, difficult book of the Fast Track series. Thanks again to the staff at PasTest for their unending patience and support in this venture. And, as always, to my folks for your support through the hard times.

AT

For Joanna (as always)

MR

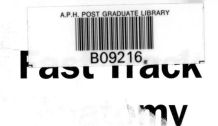

Fast Track Anatomy for

Medical Students

by

James S Taylor BSc(Hons), MBBS, MRCS
Senior House Officer Urology, Brighton & Sussex University Hospitals

Aaron Trinidade MBBR, MRCS(Ed), DO-HNS PGDipMedEd
Senior House Officer in Otolaryngology, The Royal National Throat, Nose & Ear Hospital, London

Manoj Ramachandran BSc(Hons), MBBS(Hons), MRCS(Eng), FRCS(Tr&Orth)
Consultant Paediatric and Young Adult Trauma and Orthopaedic Surgeon, Barts and the London NHS Trust, London, England and Honorary Senior Lecturer, Queen Mary's School of Medicine and Dentristry, University of London

PasTest
Dedicated to your success

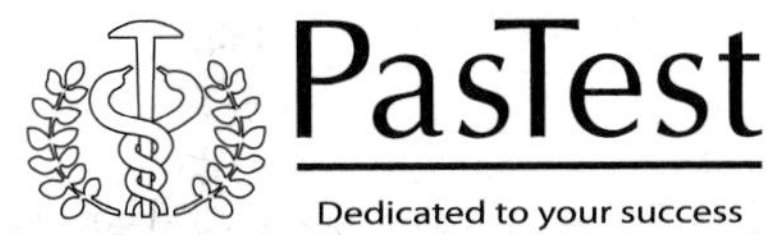

© 2008 PASTEST LTD
Egerton Court
Parkgate Estate
Knutsford
Cheshire
WA16 8DX

Telephone: 01565 752000

First Published 2008

ISBN: 1 905635 12 5
978 1 905635 12 2

A catalogue record for this book is available from the British Library.

PasTest Revision Books and Intensive Courses

PasTest has been established in the field of postgraduate medical education since 1972, providing revision books and intensive study courses for doctors preparing for their professional examinations.

Books and courses are available for the following specialties:

MRCGP, MRCP Parts 1 and 2, MRCPCH Parts 1 and 2, MRCS, MRCOG Parts 1 and 2, DRCOG, DCH, FRCA, PLAB Parts 1 and 2, Dentistry.

For further details contact:

PasTest, Freepost, Knutsford, Cheshire WA16 7BR
Tel: 01565 752000   Fax: 01565 650264
www.pastest.co.uk   enquiries@pastest.co.uk

Text prepared by Type Study, Scarborough, North Yorkshire
Printed and bound in the UK by MPG Books Ltd, Bodmin, Cornwall

INTRODUCTION

Anatomy is usually seen as one of the more tedious of the preclinical disciplines: an endless barrage of facts, lists and relations. In part, this is unfortunately true. However, by keeping the clinical importance of such tedium in mind, anatomy can become a fascinating field. It is the bread and butter of all surgical disciplines (ask any surgeon who quizzes juniors in the operating theatre!), and is also important in the procedural aspects of internal medicine.

This book deals mainly with gross anatomy. It is by no means a complete text of anatomy, but should be used in conjunction with your standard texts. It is subdivided into systems and therefore conforms to the way in which anatomy is now taught in most medical schools. The questions are based around what questions we, the authors, think you are most likely to be asked during your training and examinations (questions we ourselves were asked at some point). The layout is in two columns to allow you to cover the answers during revision. The factual aspects are for the most part presented in tabular format, a format long loved by those crammers out there! Mnemonics are used liberally, and figures are included to illustrate the more important concepts.

As always, we are keen to hear your questions/comments/corrections. It is the knowledge we gain from your contributions that help make the Fast Track series the success that it is.

JST
AT
MR

CONTRIBUTORS

Pervinder Bhogal, BSc(Hons) Neuroscience MBBS(Hons) London
Registrar in Radiology, Royal Free Hospital, London

Maninder Bhogal, BSc(Hons) Neuroscience MBBS(Hons) London
Registrar in Ophthalmology, University College Hospital, London

Benjamin Hudson, MBBS
Senior House Officer in Orthopaedics and General Surgery,
Royal Hampshire County Hospital, Winchester

Jai Kumar, BSc MBBS(Hons)
Orthopaedic Registrar, Royal Newcastle Centre, Newcastle, NSW,
Australia

Isioma Obuaya, BSc MBBS
GP Registrar, Ashley Medical Practice, Walton-on-Thames, Surrey

LIST OF TABLES

LIST OF FIGURES

CHAPTER 1: HEAD AND NECK

SURFACE MARKINGS

At what cervical level does the hyoid bone lie?	C3.
At what level does the upper border of the thyroid cartilage lie?	C4.
At what level does the cricoid cartilage lie?	C6.
What other important structure lies at the level of C4?	The bifurcation of the common carotid artery into internal and external carotid arteries.
What other important structures lie at the level of C6?	The junction of the larynx and trachea. The junction of the pharynx and oesophagus. The vertebral arteries enter the foramen transversum of C6.

ARTERIES OF THE HEAD AND NECK

How many branches does the internal carotid artery give off in the neck?	None.
How does the internal carotid artery enter the skull?	It enters the carotid canal, turns and runs forwards and medially within the temporal bone, and enters the intracranial cavity through the foramen lacerum.
What are the main branches of the internal carotid in the skull?	Anterior cerebral artery. Middle cerebral artery. Ophthalmic artery. Also branches to the middle ear, striate, hypophysis and choroid of the eye.

Of what are the posterior cerebral arteries a branch?

The basilar artery.

What are the branches of the vertebral artery?

Basilar:
- cerebellar
- pontine
- posterior cerebral.

Anterior spinal.

Which arterial system is involved in a cerebral infarct?

The internal carotid system.

Which arterial system is involved in a brainstem infarct?

The vertebral system.

Which artery is often damaged after a skull fracture and leads to an extradural haemorrhage?

The middle meningeal artery.

Of which artery is the middle meningeal artery a branch?

The maxillary artery.

Through what foramen does the middle meningeal artery enter the skull?

Foramen spinosum (it then divides into anterior and posterior branches).

What clinical finding after a head injury would suggest an extradural haemorrhage resulting from damage to the following?

Anterior branch

Hemiplegia.

Posterior branch

Deafness.

Beneath what region of the skull does the anterior branch run?

The pterion (the weakest part of the skull).

Why is knowledge about the surface markings of the anterior and posterior branches important?

These are the sites where burr holes are made to evacuate the haematoma and reduce the intracranial pressure after extradural haemorrhage.

What are the surface markings of the following?

Anterior division	3 cm above the midpoint of the zygomatic arch.
Posterior division	Where a vertical line from the mastoid process meets a horizontal line from the supraorbital margin.
What is the surface marking for the point at which the brachiocephalic trunk forms the right common carotid and right subclavian arteries?	The right sternoclavicular joint.
What are the branches of the subclavian artery?	Internal thoracic. Vertebral. Thyrocervical trunk – inferior thyroid. Suprascapular. Transverse cervical. Costocervical trunk – deep cervical. Highest intercostals.
What structure divides the subclavian artery into its three parts?	The scalenus anterior muscle (the first part is medial to, the second part beneath, the third part lateral to scalenus anterior).
How many branches come off the first part?	Three (internal thoracic, vertebral, thyrocervical trunk).
How many branches come off the second part?	One (costocervical trunk).
How many branches come off the third part?	None.
What are the nerve relations of the internal and external carotid arteries?	**Posterior:** superior laryngeal branch of vagus nerve (dividing into internal and external laryngeal nerves). **Between:** pharyngeal branch of vagus nerve, glossopharyngeal nerve. **Anterior:** hypoglossal nerve.
Which veins are used for central venous cannulation?	Internal jugular and subclavian veins.

What structure is used when measuring the jugular venous pressure (JVP)?	Internal jugular vein: the patient is placed at 45° and the height in centimetres measured from the sternal angle.
At what point does the subclavian artery become the axillary artery?	At the lateral border of the first rib.
What are the branches of the external carotid artery?	Superior thyroid artery. Ascending pharyngeal artery. Lingual artery. Facial artery. Occipital artery. Posterior auricular artery. Superficial temporal artery. Maxillary artery. (*Mnemonic:* **S**ome **A**natomists **L**ike **F**ishfingers, **O**thers **P**refer **S**ausages and **M**ash.)
How many branches does the maxillary artery usually have?	Five branches given off before the lateral pterygoid. Five branches given off within the lateral pterygoid. Five branches given off after the lateral pterygoid.
What receptors are found in the carotid arteries?	**Carotid body:** chemoreceptors. **Carotid sinus:** baroreceptors.
What lies in the carotid body?	Chemoreceptors.
What lies in the carotid sinus?	Baroreceptors.
What is the innervation of the carotid sinus and body?	Cranial nerve (CN) IX (glossopharyngeal nerve).

VEINS OF THE HEAD AND NECK

What are the surface markings of the following?

The internal jugular	Earlobe to sternoclavicular joint.
The external jugular	Earlobe to midclavicle.

What does the external jugular vein drain into?	Subclavian vein.
What is the name given to the veins within the skull?	Sinuses.
Where do the sinuses lie?	Outside the dura (between the dura and periosteum of the skull).
What is the venous drainage within the skull?	The inferior and superior petrosal sinuses: cavernous sinus superior ophthalmic vein intervenous sinus. Transverse sinus: straight sinus inferior sagittal sinus great cerebral vein. Superior sagittal sinus.
What is the lymphatic drainage of the scalp?	Occipital. Mastoid. Superficial cervical. Parotid. Submandibular. Submental. Deep nodes distributed over the course of the internal jugular vein.
Where does the superior sagittal sinus lie?	Between the two layers of falx cerebri, along the convexity of its attached margin.
Where does the inferior sagittal sinus lie?	Between the folds of the free margin of falx cerebri.
Where does the straight sinus lie?	Between the folds of the fibrous dura at the junction of falx cerebri and tentorium cerebelli.
Through which foramen does the internal jugular vein exit the skull?	The jugular foramen.

In what structure does the internal jugular vein run?

The carotid sheath.

In what structure does the external jugular vein run?

The superficial fascia of the neck.

NECK FASCIAE

What runs in the carotid sheath?

Internal carotid artery.
Internal jugular vein.
Vagus nerve.
Ansa cervicalis (wrapped around the internal jugular vein).
CNs IX, X and XII run in the upper portion of the sheath.

Which glands are located within the pretracheal fascia?

Thyroid and parathyroid glands.

What does the prevertebral fascia enclose?

Prevertebral muscles.
Vertebrae.
Errector spinae muscles.
Sympathetic trunk.
Forms the axillary sheath.

What are the attachments of the prevertebral fascia?

Cricoid cartilage and larynx.
Body of T3.
Lower border of scalenus anterior.
Third part of the subclavian artery.
This is clinically important: knowing that the thyroid gland rises on swallowing.

What is the clinical significance of the prevertebral space?

It allows infections of the neck to track down to the axilla.

FASCIAL COMPARTMENTS IN THE NECK

What are the attachments of the pretracheal fascia?

Hyoid bone.
Oblique line on thyroid cartilage.
Pericardium.
Arch of the aorta.
Carotid sheath.

Which gland is located within the pretracheal fascia?

Thyroid gland.

What are the attachments of the prevertebral fascia?

Base of the skull.
Body of T3.
Lower border of scalenus anterior.
Third part of the subclavian artery.

What is the clinical significance of the prevertebral space?

It allows infections of the neck to track down to the axilla.

What is the clinical significance of the parapharyngeal space?

This is a potential space immediately lateral to the oro- and nasopharynx. The styloid process divides it into anterior and posterior compartments. Infection here can spread to the carotid sheath, which lies in the posterior compartment.

And the retropharyngeal space?

Infection can spread from here to the posterior compartment of the parapharyngeal space and affect the **carotid sheath** as well.

And the submandibular space?

Infection here causes Ludwig's angina, a potentially airway-compromising condition.

What fascial layers are there in the neck?

Superficial.
Carotid sheath.
Prevertebral.
Pretracheal.

What is the superficial fascia?

It is a layer of connective tissue lying just deep to the platysma muscle encompassing the whole neck. This layer splits to enclose the sternocleidomastoid and trapezius muscles, parotid and submandibular glands.

In what structure does the external jugular vein run?

The superficial fascia of the neck.

Within the carotid sheath, where does the vagus nerve lie?

Between the internal jugular vein and the internal/common carotid artery.

ANTERIOR TRIANGLE OF THE NECK

What are the borders of the anterior triangle?

Lower border of the mandible.
Anterior border of the sternocleidomastoid muscle.
Midline.

What are the contents of the anterior triangle?

Arteries: common carotid artery, branches of the external carotid artery.
Veins: internal jugular, external jugular, anterior jugular veins.
Nerves: vagus, hypoglossal, nerve to mylohyoid, ansa cervicalis.
Midline structures: hyoid, larynx, trachea, oesophagus.
Muscles: strap muscles, mylohyoid, digastric, stylohyoid, geniohyoid.
Lymph nodes: submandibular, submental, anterior cervical.
Glands: thyroid, parathyroids, submandibular.

What are the causes of a lump in the anterior or posterior triangles?

Lymph nodes.
Salivary glands – submandibular and parotid gland (anterior) and ranulae.
Skin lumps.
Cystic structures – branchial (anterior), cystic hygroma (posterior).
Vascular – carotid body tumour, aneurysm.

What is a cystic hygroma?

Cystic hygromas are multiloculated cystic structures that are benign in nature. They form as a result of budding lymphatics. Failure to establish venous drainage results in dilated, disorganised lymph channels, which, in the largest form, present as cystic hygromas, usually in childhood.

What is a ranula?

A pseudocyst that is associated with mucus extravasation into the surrounding soft tissues, resulting from trauma to the salivary gland excretory duct. Obstruction of salivary flow is implicated in some instances.

POSTERIOR TRIANGLE OF THE NECK

What are the boundaries of the posterior triangle?

Posterior border of sternocleidomastoid.
Anterior border of trapezius.
Medial two-thirds of the clavicle.

What forms the floor of the posterior triangle?

Semispinalis capitus.
Splenius capitus.
Scalenus anterior, medius and posterior.
Serratus anterior.
(All covered by prevertebral fascia.)

What are the contents of the posterior triangle?

Arteries: transverse cervical, suprascapular of the thyrocervical trunk, subclavian.
Veins: transverse cervical, suprascapular, external jugular, subclavian.
Nerves: branches of the cervical plexus, spinal accessory, trunks of brachial plexus, phrenic.
Muscles: omohyoid.
Lymphatics: occipital, supraclavicular.

HYOID BONE AND THE STRAP MUSCLES

What are the attachments of the hyoid bone?

Suprahyoid:
- middle constrictor
- ligament of stylohyoid
- hyoglossus
- genioglossus
- mylohyoid.

Infrahyoid:
- thyrohyoid membrane
- strap muscles.

From which pharyngeal arch is the hyoid derived?

Second forms the lesser cornu and superior body.
Third forms the greater cornu and inferior body.

What are the strap muscles?

Sternohyoid.
Thyrohyoid.
Sternothyroid.
Omohyoid.
(Also known as infrahyoid muscles)

What is the nerve supply of the strap muscles?

Ansa cervicalis.

What is the function of the strap muscles?

They depress the hyoid bone and larynx during phonation.

What is the function of the suprahyoid muscles?

Raise the hyoid bone, thereby raising the floor of the mouth and pressing the tongue against the hard palate.

What is the ansa cervicalis?

It is formed from the cervical nerves. The loop is completed by the superior (C1) root and inferior (C2 + C3) roots forming a loop. C1 temporarily joins the hypoglossal nerve. The loop supplies the infrahyoid muscles.

THORACIC INLET

What are the margins of the thoracic inlet?

The **superior thoracic aperture** (as it is also called) is bounded by: the first thoracic vertebra (T1) *posteriorly*, the first pair of ribs *laterally* (more specifically, the first ribs form lateral C-shaped curves posterior to anterior) and the superior border of the manubrium *anteriorly*.

What passes through the thoracic inlet?

Trachea.
Oesophagus.
Nerves:
- phrenic nerve
- vagus nerve
- recurrent laryngeal nerves
- sympathetic trunks.

Arteries:
- common carotid arteries
- brachiocephalic trunk
- subclavian arteries.

Veins:
- internal jugular veins
- brachiocephalic veins
- subclavian veins.

Lymph nodes and lymphatic vessels.

How many cervical sympathetic ganglia are there?

Superior, middle and cervicothoracic or stellate ganglia.

How are the sympathetic nerves distributed?

On the surface of blood vessels from the sympathetic trunk, because no sympathetic nerves arise from above T1.

What is Horner's syndrome?

Loss of sympathetic supply to the face as a result of an interruption of the sympathetic nerve supply. The interruption can occur as a result of a tumour invading the trunk (Pancoast's tumour), avulsion of thoracic roots (brachial plexus injuries) or high thoracic spinal cord injuries. The signs are unilateral, with a flushed, dry face and a small pupil with ptosis (drooping) of the upper eyelid.

What are the branches of the cervical plexus?

Lesser occipital (C2).
Great auricular (C2 + C3).
Transverse cervical (C2 + C3).
Supraclavicular (C3 + C4).
They supply the cutaneous distribution of part of the neck.

LYMPH SYSTEM OF THE HEAD AND NECK

Name the cervical lymph nodes

Rings:
- submental
- submandibular
- preauricular
- postauricular
- occipital.

Chains:
- superficial
- deep (jugulo-digastric, jugulo-omohyoid, retropharyngeal, paratracheal).

What is important about the lymphatic drainage of the tongue?

There is crossover so that lymph drains to nodes bilaterally.

Into where does the thoracic duct drain?

The junction of the left subclavian vein and the left internal jugular vein.

From which region does lymph drain into the thoracic duct?

Both sides below the diaphragm. The left side of the head, neck and thorax.

Into where does lymph from the right side of the head, neck and thorax drain?

The right lymphatic duct, which then drains into the venous system at the junction of the right subclavian vein and the right internal jugular vein.

CRANIAL NERVES

What is the nerve supply to the muscles of facial expression?

Facial nerve (except levator palpebrae superioris – supplied by CN III).

What is the nerve supply to the muscles of mastication?

The trigeminal nerve V3 (except buccinator – supplied by CN VII).

What is the sensory supply to the face?

Trigeminal nerve.

What is the part of the face not supplied by this nerve?

The angle of the jaw.

Which nerve supplies the muscles of the pharynx and palate?

Pharyngeal plexus, CNs IX and X, sympathetics (except stylopharyngeus, which is supplied by CN IX and the medial pterygoid, which is supplied by CN V3).

Which nerve supplies the muscles of the tongue?

CN XII (except palatoglossus which is supplied by CNs IX and X), sympathetics and the pharyngeal plexus.

Which nerve supplies the larynx?

Recurrent laryngeal nerve (except cricothyroid – supplied by superior laryngeal nerve).

What obvious clinical findings are present in a trigeminal nerve lesion?

Jaw deviation towards the lesion.
Weakness of the masseters and temporalis muscles on the affected side.
Sensory loss to the area affected.
Decreased or absent corneal reflex on the side of the lesion.

How does facial expression differ in UMN and LMN lesions of the facial nerve?

The facial nuclei receive supranuclear input from the cerebral hemispheres. This input is mainly to the part of the facial nucleus that supplies the frontalis muscle and it is bilateral. There is no bilateral input from the hemispheres to the part of the nucleus supplying the lower part of the face. Therefore, in unilateral UMN (upper motor neurone) lesions of the facial nerve the frontalis is spared and only the lower part of the face is affected – the patient can still furrow the brow. In unilateral LMN (lower motor neurone) facial nerve lesions all the muscles are affected.

How can the signs help determine the site of the lesion?

The long complicated course and multiple branches make damage at numerous levels possible.

Pons: the nerve encircles the nucleus of the abducent nerve in the pons. A lesion that affects both the muscles of the face and the lateral rectus would imply damage at the level of the pons.

Cerebellopontine angle: at this site the cranial nerves V, VI, VII and VIII are in close apposition. Damage at this site would affect these nerves also.

Petrous temporal bone: the nerve traverses the petrous temporal bone via the facial canal. As it traverses this canal, fibres are given off for taste (chorda tympani) and to the stapedius muscle. Lesions can thus cause a loss of taste on the anterior two-thirds of the tongue and hyperacusis as a result of loss of muscle control to the stapedius muscle.

In the face: the nerve passes through the parotid gland and gives off multiple branches at this level. Here it is liable to damage from trauma, parotid gland disease, etc.

Can patients with hemiplegia still have emotional facial responses?

Yes. They may still be able to laugh or smile, etc. It is believed that the fibres controlling mimetic movements run a separate course to the main corticobulbar fibres and these may be spared. In extensive lesions, however, sparing is unlikely.

What is Bell's palsy?

Bell's palsy is a form of temporary facial paralysis resulting from infection or trauma to the facial nerve. It is the most common cause of facial paralysis. The symptoms begin suddenly and reach their peak within 48 hours. It is believed to have a viral cause, either herpes simplex or a meningitis virus. The facial nerve swells and becomes inflamed in reaction to the infection.

What is Ramsay Hunt syndrome?

A LMN facial nerve palsy caused by the varicella-zoster virus. It is characterised by several crusted lesions and blisters in the left external acoustic meatus and pinna (zoster oticus) behind the ear on the mastoid process, as well as the anterior two-thirds of the tongue and hard and soft palate. The lesions are almost always unilateral and on the same side as the facial palsy. Ramsay Hunt hypothesised that patients formerly infected with varicella (chickenpox) could have a reactivation of latent virus that had laid dormant in the geniculate ganglion of the facial nerve.

Where does the spinal accessory and cervical plexus emerge?

At the midpoint of the posterior border of the sternocleidomastoid muscle.

What are the branches of the facial nerve given off within the parotid?

Temporal.
Zygomatic.
Buccal.
Mandibular.
Cervical.

(*Mnemonic:* **T**en **Z**ulus **B**uried **M**y **C**at.)

Which branches are given off before the parotid?

Greater petrosal nerve.
Chorda tympani.
Nerve to posterior belly of digastric.
Nerve to stylohyoid.

What is the function of buccinator?

It helps return food from the cheeks to the mouth during chewing.

Is there a cranial root to nerve XI?

It was believed that that this nerve had both a cranial and a spinal root. It has been shown, however, that the cranial root is actually part of the vagus nerve.

Is the nerve liable to damage?

The nerve can easily be damaged in several procedures. Its course lies in close proximity to the internal carotid artery so it can be easily damaged during carotid endarterectomy or central line insertion. It also has an almost subcutaneous route in the posterior triangle, so it can be damaged through trauma or procedures such as lymph node biopsy.

What signs would you see if it was damaged?

Drooping of the shoulder.
Difficulty in raising the arm above the horizontal on the affected side.
Difficulty/inability to turn the head away from the side of the lesion.

TEMPOROMANDIBULAR JOINT

What type of joint is the temporomandibular joint (TMJ)?

Atypical synovial joint.
Condyloid.

What is the nerve supply of the TMJ?

Auriculotemporal nerve and the nerve to masseter.

Which bone is the 'socket' part of?	The squamous part of the temporal bone.
Which muscles cause opening of the mouth?	Lateral pterygoid. Digastric.
Which muscles cause closing of the mouth?	Masseter. Medial pterygoid. Temporalis.
Which muscle causes protraction of the mandible?	Lateral pterygoid.
What muscle causes retraction of the mandible?	Temporalis.
What is the TMJ?	A synovial joint between the condylar head of the mandible and the articular tubercle on the squamous part of the temporal bone. The articular surfaces are covered with an articular cartilage and divided by an articular disc.
How does it function?	The condylar articular surface slides forwards from the mandibular fossa of the temporal bone to the articular tubercle.

INFRATEMPORAL FOSSA AND PTERYGOPALATINE FOSSAE

Where is the infratemporal fossa?	It lies between the base of the skull, pharynx and mandible.
What are its boundaries?	It is bounded by the following structures: **anteriorly** by the infratemporal surface of the maxilla and the ridge, which descends from its zygomatic process **posteriorly** by the articular tubercle of the temporal and the spinal angularis of the sphenoid **superiorly** by the great wing of the sphenoid below the

infratemporal crest, and by the undersurface of the temporal squama
inferiorly by the alveolar border of the maxilla
medially by the lateral pterygoid plate.

What occupies the temporal and infratemporal fossa?

Muscles of mastication (temporalis. [lower part], internal and external pterygoids)
Maxillary artery.
Mandibular nerve.
Otic ganglion.
Chorda tympani nerve.

PTERYGOPALATINE FOSSA

What are the contents of the pterygopalatine fossa?

Terminal branches of the maxillary artery.
Maxillary division of the trigeminal nerve.
The pteryopalatine ganglion.

Where is the pterygomaxillary fissure?

Between the lateral pterygoid plate and the maxilla. Deep to this lies the pterygopalatine fossa.

What are the contents of the pterygopalatine fossa?

Terminal branches of the maxillary artery.
Maxillary division of the trigeminal nerve.
The pteryopalatine ganglion (nerve of the pterygoid canal – formed by the fusion of the deep petrosal nerve, sympathetic and greater petrosal nerve, parasympathetic from facial nerve).

Where does the pterygopalatine fossa lie?

Anterior to the pterygoid plates of the sphenoid and posterior to the maxilla and lateral to the perpendicular plate of the palatine bone.

What does the pterygopalatine ganglion contain?

Greater petrosal nerve: postganglionic parasympathetic nerves – branch of facial nerve at petrous part of temporal bone. Secretomotor action.
Deep petrosal nerve: sympathetic nerves – from carotid plexus via internal carotid artery. Vasomotor action.
Nerve of pterygoid canal: joined greater petrosal and deep petrosal nerves.
Maxillary nerve: sensory.

What does the pterygopalatine ganglion supply?

Nose, nasopharynx and palate: the nerves produced by the pterygopalatine ganglion include:

- the greater palatine nerve (mucous membrane of palate and gums)
- posteroinferior nasal branches (lateral wall of nose)
- lesser palatine nerves (soft palate and tonsilar region)
- posterosuperior nasal nerves (lateral wall of nasal cavity and septum via nasopalatine nerve)
- pharyngeal (nasopharynx).

SKULL SINUSES

What are the various air sinuses of the skull?

Frontal, draining to the middle meatus.
Ethmoid, draining to middle and superior meatuses.
Maxillary, draining to hiatus semilunaris in the middle meatus.
Spenoidal, draining to the sphenoethmoidal recess above superior concha.
Cavernous sinus.

What are the functions of the sinuses?	To lighten the skull. To resonate the voice. To moisten air.
Which pair of sinuses is not present at birth?	The frontal sinuses (appear at around age 2).
Which sinus may give surgical access to the pituitary gland?	Sphenoid sinus.
What are the parts of the mandible?	Body. Vertical ramus. Angle of mandible. Anterior pointed coronoid process. Posterior rounded condylar process.
Where is the mental foramen?	It lies between the roots of the fifth and sixth lower teeth (between the second premolar and first molar).
What is the function of the buccinator muscle?	It helps return food from the cheeks to the mouth during chewing.
In which intracranial fossa does the cavernous sinus lie?	Middle cranial fossa.
Which structures run in the lateral wall of the cavernous sinus?	CNs III, IV, Va, Vb.
Which structures run in the roof of the cavernous sinus?	Middle cerebral artery. CN II.
Which structures run within the cavernous sinus?	CN VI. Internal carotid artery.
Which structures are medial to the cavernous sinus?	Pituitary fossa and gland within it. Sphenoid sinus.
What is the main cause of cavernous sinus thrombosis?	Infection of the facial skin.
Why?	Part of the venous drainage from the face is through the orbit and into the cavernous sinus.

What are the clinical signs of cavernous sinus thrombosis?
Ophthalmoplegia.
Chemosis.
Pain.

Where does the temporalis muscle insert?
Onto the coronoid process of the mandible.

How can you test the function of the glossopharyngeal nerve?
Check taste sensation.
Check the gag reflex – lost on the ipsilateral side of a lesion.

SALIVARY GLANDS

What are the three main salivary glands?
Parotid – serous.
Submandibular – mixed mucous and serous.
Sublingual – mucous.

What nerve causes the secretion of saliva in the parotid?
Via the postganglionic parasympathetic fibres, arriving via the otic ganglion and then the auriculotemporal nerve.

What structure splits the parotid into its superficial and deep parts?
The branches of the facial nerve.

What are the boundaries of the parotid gland?
Anterior:
ramus of mandible
masseter.
Posterior:
sternocleidomastoid.
Deep:
zygomatic arch
posterior belly of digastric muscle.
Superficial:
platysma muscle
skin.
Superior:
cartilaginous part of external acoustic meatus
TMJ.
Inferior:
border of mandible.

Why is gland swelling painful?
Thought to be caused by pressure as a result of swelling contained within the sheath; a continuation of the superficial fascial sheath.

What structures are found within the gland?
Retromandibular vein.
External carotid.
Parotid lymph nodes.
Auriculotemporal nerve (mandibular).

Where does the parotid duct enter the mouth?
Stenson's duct passes anterior to the masseter, entering opposite the upper second molar teeth. It runs in the line between the tragus and the nostril.

What is the lymphatic drainage?
Nodes from the superficial and deep surfaces drain to cervical nodes.

What is Frey's syndrome and why does it occur?
When there is stimulation of saliva secretion there is sweating of the cheek. It occurs when there is regrowth of parasympathetic fibres into damaged sympathetic fibres of the auriculotemporal nerve (usually a result of parotid surgery).

What are the parts of the submandibular gland?
Superficial: larger part lying superficial to the mylohyoid muscle.
Deep: smaller part deep to this muscle. The two parts are continuous posterior to this muscle.

Where does the gland lie?
Superficial: laterally against the inner surface of the mandible in the shallow mandibular fossa.
Deep: deep to the mylohoid muscle but superficial to the hyoglossus muscle.

What are the nerves associated with the deep part of the submandibular gland?
The lingual nerve runs above it giving rise to the submandibular ganglion. The hypoglossal nerve runs below it.

What are the vessels related to the superficial part?

Facial artery: over upper border of gland.
Facial vein: over the lateral superficial surface.

Where does its duct enter the mouth?

At the sublingual papilla beside the frenulum after running a course on the surface of the hyoglossus, passing between the sublingual gland and the genioglossus muscle.

What is another name for the submandibular duct?

Wharton's duct.

Which nerve is closely related to the duct?

Lingual nerve (mandibular joined by chorda tympanic branch of facial). It crosses the duct laterally and superficially, and ascends on the medial side of the duct, supplying the anterior two-thirds of the tongue.

Where does the sublingual gland lie?

It is a superficial structure in the floor of the mouth between the mucous membrane and the anterior part of the mylohyoid muscle. Laterally it lies against the mandible.

Where do the ducts open?

The multiple small ducts open at the sublingual fold.

What is Ludwig's angina?

A submandibular or sublingual space infection. It is a type of cellulitis that involves inflammation of the tissues of the floor of the mouth, under the tongue. It often occurs after an infection of the roots of the teeth or a mouth injury. Swelling of the tissues occurs rapidly and may block the airway or prevent swallowing of saliva.

PHARYNX AND LARYNX

What is the pharynx?	A fibromuscular tube applied to the base of the skull with an inferior opening continuous with the oesophagus and trachea.
What are the parts of the pharynx?	It lies behind the nasal cavity, oral cavity and the larynx so is called the nasopharynx, oropharynx and the laryngopharynx.
What are the layers of the pharynx?	Stratified squamous epithelium, pharyngobasilar fascia, muscular layer, buccopharyngeal fascia.
From which pharyngeal arch is the larynx derived?	Fourth and sixth.
What are the muscles of the pharynx?	Superior, middle and inferior constrictor muscles, all overlapping posteriorly. The lower muscle lies outside the upper.
What structures pass between the superior and middle constrictors?	Glossopharyngeal nerve. Stylopharyngeus muscle. Stylohyoid ligament. Lingual nerve.
Where does a pharyngeal pouch (dehiscence of Killian) form?	Between thyropharyngeus and cricopharyngeus (the upper and lower parts of the inferior constrictor respectively). It is a diverticulum in which food boluses can lodge, leading to perforation.
What are the boundaries of the retropharyngeal space?	This space is limited above by the base of the skull, while below it extends behind the oesophagus into the posterior mediastinal cavity of the thorax.
What is the vallecula?	This is the midline fold between the tongue and epiglottis. An important landmark in intubation.

What is the blood supply of the larynx?

Superior and inferior laryngeal arteries.
Ascending pharyngeal artery.
Facial artery.
Lingual artery.
Inferior thyroid artery.

What is the sensory supply to the larynx?

Internal branch of the superior laryngeal nerve (vagus) above the vocal folds.
Recurrent laryngeal nerve (vagus) below the larynx.

Where does the recurrent laryngeal nerve enter the larynx?

Below the lower border of the inferior constrictor.

How can one remember the various derivatives of the branchial arches?

(*Mnemonic:* **M**uscles **S**upport the **P**harynx and **L**arynx.)
First arch (**m**andibular arch; also known as **M**eckel's cartilage):

- **m**uscles of mastication
- **m**andible
- **m**andibular nerve (CN V3)
- **m**ucous membrane (anterior two-thirds of tongue)
- **m**axillary artery.

Second arch (hyoid arch):

- **s**tapes
- **s**tyloid process
- **s**tylohyoid ligament
- **s**uperior part and lesser cornu of hyoid bone
- **s**miling muscles (of facial expression) and their nervous system (CN VII).

Third arch:

- stylo**p**haryngeus and glosso**p**haryngeus muscles
- inferior part and greater cornu of hyoid bone.

Fourth and sixth arches:
- **p**haryngeal and **l**aryngeal parts of the vagus nerve (CN X)
- cartilages of the **l**arynx: thyroid, cricoids, arytenoids, epiglottis
- muscles of the **l**arynx.

Fifth arch:
- no derivatives.

What is deglutition?

Swallowing: divided into a voluntary phase consisting of preparing the food bolus and moving it to the oropharynx, and an involuntary phase that involves elevation of the soft palate, depressing the epiglottis and larynx, and successive contractions of the pharyngeal constrictors to allow the food bolus to enter the oesophagus.

What nerves are involved with deglutition?

Glossopharyngeal and vagus nerves.

What is a bulbar palsy?

Bilateral motor nuclei impairment of CNs IX, X and XII resulting in dysphagia (difficulty in swallowing), dysphonia and poor cough reflex.

What is the larynx?

It has two features: it acts as a sphincter to separate the respiratory from the alimentary tract; the second is an adaptation for phonation. It consists of cartilages, membranes and muscles, and is continuous superiorly with the laryngopharynx and inferiorly with the trachea.

What is the function of the larynx?

Prevents aspiration during swallowing.
Phonation.
Coughing.
Straining (the Valsalva manoeuvre).

What are the cartilages of the larynx?

Epiglottis: elastic cartilage.
Thyroid: hyaline cartilage.

Arytenoid: hyaline cartilage.
Cricoid: hyaline cartilage.

What is the lymphatic drainage of the larynx?

To the deep cervical nodes.

Where is the epiglottis attached?

Inferiorly it is attached to the internal aspect of the anterior upper thyroid. The proximal portion projects above the hyoid bone. It covers the larynx on deglutition.

What are the vocal folds made from?

They are the free upper border of the cricothyroid membrane. It joins the arytenoid cartilage posteriorly to the thyroid cartilage anteriorly.

What are the vestibular ligaments?

The lower free border of the quadrangular membrane forms this ligament. This less distinct membrane joins the arytenoid cartilages to the epiglottis.

What is the rima glottidis?

The space between the vocal folds.

What are the functions of the intrinsic and extrinsic muscles of the larynx?

Extrinsic: stabilise or move the larynx as a whole. They raise the larynx on swallowing.
Intrinsic: alter the position of one part. They protect the airway and adjust the vocal ligaments for phonation.

What are the laryngeal muscles?

Intrinsic:
- cricothyroid
- posterior cricoarytenoid
- lateral cricoarytenoid
- transverse arytenoids
- thyroarytenoid
- oblique arytenoids.

Extrinsic:
- digastric
- mylohyoid
- stylohyoid
- geniohyoid

stylopharyngeus
palatopharyngeus
strap muscles.

What is the internal laryngeal muscle nerve supply?

The recurrent laryngeal nerve of the vagus nerve supplies all the intrinsic muscles, except the cricothyroid muscle (external laryngeal nerve of the superior laryngeal nerve of the vagus).

Which intrinsic laryngeal muscles close the folds?

Oblique arytenoids.
Transverse arytenoids.
Lateral cricoarytenoid.

Which intrinsic muscle opens the vocal folds?

Posterior cricoarytenoid: the implications for paralysis of this muscle is an obstructed airway.

Which intrinsic muscle tightens the cord?

Cricothyroid.

What is the nerve supply of the mucous membrane of the larynx?

Internal laryngeal nerve (of the superior laryngeal nerve of the vagus) supplies the membrane above the vocal folds. It is accompanied by the superior laryngeal artery (of the superior thyroid artery of the external carotid).
Recurrent laryngeal nerve (of the vagus nerve) supplies the membrane below the folds. It is accompanied by the inferior thyroid artery of the thyrocervical trunk of the subclavian artery.

Which common operations risk damage to the recurrent laryngeal nerve?

Thyroidectomy and parathyroidectomy.

What is Semon's law?

Transection of the recurrent laryngeal nerve causes complete paralysis (folds half abducted/adducted). Trauma to the nerve causes partial paralysis (folds adducted).

Why is this important?	If there is trauma to the nerves bilaterally both folds are adducted and the patient's airway is obstructed and he or she cannot breathe.
How can the vagus be tested?	The vagus is involved in the efferent pathway of the gag reflex along with the glossopharyngeal nerve. Innervation of the soft palate can be tested by asking the patient to say 'Ah'. This tests the muscles of the soft palate and the uvula should rise. Lesions of the nerve will cause the uvula to deviate AWAY from the side of the lesion.

PALATINE TONSILS

What forms the anterior and posterior palatine pillars?	Anterior: palatoglossus. Posterior: palatopharyngeus. The tonsils lie within the fold formed.
What forms the lateral wall of the tonsillar fossa?	Superior constrictor.
What is the arterial supply of the palatine tonsils?	Ascending palatine artery (facial, external carotid). Tonsillar branch (facial, external carotid).
What is Waldeyer's ring?	An interrupted circle of lymphoid tissue in the pharynx.
What important structure runs posterolateral to the tonsillar fossa?	The carotid sheath and the structures within it.

PALATE

What bones make up the hard palate?	Palatine process of the maxilla. Horizontal plate of the palatine bone.
What is the blood supply to the hard palate?	Greater palatine artery.

What muscles form the soft palate?

Tensor veli palatini: mandibular nerve.
Levator veli palatini: vagus nerve.
Muscles of the uvula: vagus nerve.
Palatoglossus: vagus nerve.
Palatopharyngeus: vagus nerve.

What is the function of the soft palate?

To close the nasopharynx (e.g. during swallowing, to prevent regurgitation of food into the nose).

What is the uvula?

The midline projection at the posterior border of the soft palate. It can be easily visualised in an open mouth.

TRACHEA

What is a cricothyroidotomy or tracheostomy?

An emergency puncture of the cricothyroid membrane to insert an airway. A tracheostomy is a surgical procedure involving an incision into the trachea creating a temporary or permanent airway.

What are the landmarks of the trachea?

Commences at cricoid cartilage (C6), bifurcating at C4–5. It is approximately 10 cm in length.

What is its structure?

Incomplete C-shaped hyaline cartilage rings completed posteriorly by the smooth muscle trachealis. Membranes connect each ring.

Table 1.1 Muscles of facial expression

Muscle	Origin	Route	Insertion	Action	Innervation
Orbicularis oculi 1. Inner palpebral part 2. Outer orbital part 3. Lacrimal part	1. Medial palpebral ligament 2. Lateral palpebral raphe 3. Frontal bone, maxilla (orbital medial margin) Lacrimal bone	1. Fibres travel within upper and lower eyelids 2. Fibres loop around orbital margin 3. Fibres pass deep to lacrimal sac	1. Medial palpebral ligament 2. Lateral palpebral raphe. Insertion into origin 3. Lateral palpebral raphe	1. Close the palpebral fissure gently. Allows blinking 2. Close palpebral fissure tightly – 'screwing up eyes' 3. Dilate lacrimal sac, enhancing tear drainage	Temporal branch of facial n. Zygomatic branch of facial n.
Levator palpebrae superioris	Inferior surface of lesser wing of sphenoid	Fibres enter upper eyelid	Upper part of tarsal plate	Raise upper eyelid	Voluntary fibres from oculomotor n. Involuntary fibres from sympathetic neurons
Corrugator supercilii	Medial end of superciliary arch	Fibres pass upwards and laterally between palpebral and orbital portions of orbicularis oculi	Deep surface of the skin above middle of the orbital arch	Draws eyebrows downwards and medially – 'wrinkles forehead' in frowning	Temporal branch of facial n.
Procerus	Fascia covering lower part of nasal bone and lateral nasal cartilage	Fibres travel upwards and decussate with those of frontalis	Skin between eyebrows	Draws down skin over medial part of eyebrows – 'wrinkling nose'	Buccal branch of facial n.

Table 1.1 Muscles of facial expression (continued)

Muscle	Origin	Route	Insertion	Action	Innervation
Nasalis 1. Transverse part 2. Alar part	1. Middle of maxilla 2. Greater alar cartilage	1. Fibres travel upwards and medially, expanding into thin aponeurosis 2. Fibres travel directly	1. Transverse part on opposite side 2. Skin at point of nose	Maintain opening of external nares during forceful inspiration	Buccal branch of facial n.
Depressor septi	Incisive fossa of maxilla	Fibres ascend	Nasal septum and ala	Draws nasal ala downwards, constricting nares	Buccal branches of facial n.
Orbicularis oris 1. Lateral band 2. Medial band 3. Inferior portion	1. Alveolar border of maxilla 2. Nasal septum 3. Lateral to midline of mandible	Fibres sweep around the mouth	Is continuous with other muscles at angle of the mouth	Protrusion and closure of lips – 'puckering up for a kiss'	Mandibular and buccal branches of facial n.
Levator labii superioris 1. Angular head 2. Infraorbital head	1. Upper frontal process of maxilla and zygomatic bone 2. Lower margin of orbit	1. Fibres travel obliquely downwards and laterally into two slips 2. Fibres converge	1. Skin of nose, upper lip and greater alar cartilage 2. Muscles of upper lip	1. Dilates the nares and elevates the upper lip – 'snarling' 2. Elevates upper lip	Buccal branches of facial n.
Levator anguli oris	Canine fossa	Fibres travel obliquely downwards	Angle of the mouth	Elevates angle of the mouth	Buccal branches of facial n.

Table 1.1 Continued

Muscle	Origin	Route	Insertion	Action	Innervation
Zygomaticus major	Zygomatic bone	Fibres travel anteriorly downwards and medially	Angle of the mouth	Draws angle of mouth superiorly and posteriorly, used in 'smiling'	Buccal branches of facial n.
Zygomaticus minor	Zygomatic bone	Fibres travel anteriorly, inferiorly and medially	Upper lip	Elevates and everts upper lip	Buccal branches of facial n.
Risorius	Fascia overlying masseter muscle	Fibres travel horizontally forwards	Skin at angle of the mouth	Retracts angle of the mouth to produce smiling not involving skin around eyes – 'grinning'	Buccal branches of facial n.
Depressor labii inferioris	Oblique line of the mandible	Fibres travel upwards and medially	Skin of lower lip	Draws lower lip downwards and laterally	Mandibular branch of facial n.
Depressor anguli oris	Oblique line of the mandible	Fibres converge from oblique line of the mandible	Angle of the mouth	Depresses angle of the mouth – 'frowning'	Mandibular branch of facial n.
Mentalis	Incisive fossa of mandible	Fibres travel upwards and laterally	Skin of chin	Raises and protrudes lower lip – 'wrinkles chin'	Mandibular branch of facial n.

Table 1.1 Muscles of facial expression (continued)

Muscle	Origin	Route	Insertion	Action	Innervation
Buccinator	Outer surfaces of alveolar processes of the maxilla and mandible over molars and pterygomandibular raphe	The fibres converge towards the angle of the mouth, where central fibres intersect each other; upper and lower fibres continue forwards into corresponding lip without decussation	Orbicularis oris	Compresses cheek against teeth Used in blowing Empties gutter between the teeth and cheek during mastication	Buccal branches of facial n.
Epicranius 1. Occipital belly (occipitalis) 2. Frontal belly (frontalis)	1. Lateral two-thirds of superior nuchal line of occipital bone; mastoid process of temporal bone 2. Galea aponeurotica	1. Fibres sweep forwards over scalp 2. Fibres sweep forwards and medially	1. Galea aponeurotica; skin above nose and eyes 2. Fascia of facial muscles	1. Draws back scalp, aiding frontal belly to 'wrinkle forehead' and raise eyebrows 2. Draws back scalp, raises eyebrows, 'wrinkles forehead'	1. Posterior auricular n. (branch of facial artery) 2. Temporal branch of facial n.
Temporoparietalis	Fascia over ear	Fibres fan out	Lateral border of galea aponeurotica	Tightens scalp, raises ears	Temporal branch of facial n.
Auricularis 1. Anterior 2. Superior 3. Posterior	1. Galea aponeurotica anterior to ear 2. Galea aponeurotica superior to ear 3. Mastoid process		1. Anterior to ear helix 2. Superior part of ear 3. Posterior part of ear	1. Draws ear forward in some people, moves scalp 2. Draws ear upwards in some people, moves scalp 3. Draws ear upwards	1. Temporal branch of facial n. 2. Temporal branch of facial n. 3. Posterior auricular branch of facial n.

Table 1.2 Muscles of mastication

Muscle	Origin	Route	Insertion	Action	Innervation
Temporalis	Temporal fossa Temporal fascia	Fibres pass through the temporal fossa	Coronoid process of the mandible Anterior border of ramus of mandible	Closes lower jaw, clenches teeth	Mandibular division of trigeminal n.
Masseter 1. Deeper part 2. Superficial part	1. Inner surface of zygomatic arch 2. Anterior undersurface of zygomatic arch	1. Fibres run vertically downwards 2. Fibres run downwards and backwards	1. Outer aspect of ramus of mandible 2. Outer surface of ascending ramus of mandible	1. Closes lower jaw, clenches teeth 2. Superficial fibres slightly protract jaw	Mandibular division of trigeminal n.
Pterygoideus medialis (medial pterygoid)	Medial surface of lateral pterygoid plate	Fibres travel downwards, backwards and laterally	Medial surface of the angle of the mandible	Closes jaw, clenches teeth	Medial pterygoid n. (branch of mandibular division of trigeminal n.)
Pterygoideus lateralis (lateral pterygoid) 1. Superior head 2. Inferior head	1. Lateral surface of greater wing of sphenoid 2. Lateral aspect of lateral pterygoid plate	Fibres run backwards and laterally	1. Pterygoid fovea 2. Temporomandibular joint	Opens jaw, protrudes mandible, moves mandible sideways during chewing	Lateral pterygoid n. (branch of mandibular division of trigeminal n.)

Table 1.3 Muscles of the neck

Muscle	Origin	Route	Insertion	Action	Innervation
Sternocleidomastoid 1. Sternal head 2. Clavicular head	1. Anterior surface of the manubrium sterni 2. Medial third of clavicle	Fibres run posteriorly and laterally	Lateral half of occipital superior nuchal line and mastoid process	1. Lateral flexion and lateral rotation of the neck 2. Accessory muscle of respiration – both sides draw sternum superiorly in deep inspiration	Spinal part of accessory n. with sensory supply from C2, C3
Platysma	Subcutaneous fascia and skin of the chest and shoulder	Fibres sweep upwards over the front and sides of the neck	Deep fascia of the neck, lower border of the mandible and deep fascia of the lower face	Depresses and draws lower lip laterally, draws up skin of chest, depresses mandible	Cervical branch of facial n.
Digastricus 1. Anterior belly 2. Posterior belly	1. Digastric fossa of mandible 2. Mastoid notch	Bellies are united by an intermediate tendon, which slides through a small fibrous fascial sling	Fibrous sling attached to hyoid bone	1. When hyoid is fixed, depresses the mandible 2. When hyoid is unfixed, raises hyoid during swallowing	1. Mandibular division of trigeminal 2. Facial n.
Stylohyoid	Styloid process of temporal bone	Fibres split around the intermediate tendon of the digastric muscle	Hyoid bone	Elevates and retracts hyoid bone	Facial n.

Table 1.3 Continued

Muscle	**Origin**	**Route**	**Insertion**	**Action**	**Innervation**
Mylohyoid	Mylohyoid line of mandible	Fibres form a sling or diaphragm across the floor of the mouth	Body of the hyoid bone	Elevates hyoid bone, raises floor of mouth and tongue	Mylohyoid n. from inferior alveolar n., branch of mandibular division of trigeminal n.
Sternohyoid[a]	Sternal end of clavicle, posterior sternoclavicular ligament and posterior surface of manubrium	Fibres pass upwards and medially	Body of hyoid bone	Depresses hyoid bone	Ansa cervicalis (C1–3)
Sternothyroid[a]	Posterior surface of manubrium	Fibres pass upwards and medially	Oblique line on lamina of thyroid cartilage	Depresses thyroid cartilage	Ansa cervicalis (C1–3)
Thyrohyoid[a]	Oblique line of thyroid cartilage	Fibres travel upwards	Greater cornu of hyoid bone	Depresses hyoid, raises thyroid cartilage	Ansa cervicalis (C1)

Table 1.3 Muscles of the neck (continued)

Muscle	Origin	Route	Insertion	Action	Innervation
Omohyoid[a] 1. Inferior belly 2. Superior belly	1. Superior border of scapula medial to scapular notch 2. Intermediate tendon	1. Fibres incline forwards and upwards where they converge into an intermediate tendon bound to the clavicle by a fibrous expansion 2. Fibres pass almost vertically upwards close to lateral border of sternohyoid	1. Intermediate tendon 2. Lower border of hyoid bone lateral to sternohyoid insertion	1. Depresses hyoid bone, divides posterior triangle of the neck into upper/occipital triangle and lower/subclavian triangle 2. Depresses hyoid bone, divides anterior triangle of the neck into upper/carotid triangle and lower/carotid triangle	Ansa cervicalis
Longus colli 1. Superior oblique part 2. Inferior oblique part 3. Vertical part	1. Anterior tubercles of transverse processes of third, fourth and fifth cervical vertebrae 2. Anterior surfaces of first two/three thoracic vertebral bodies 3. Anterior surfaces of upper three thoracic and lower three cervical vertebral bodies	1. Fibres ascend obliquely and medially 2. Fibres ascend obliquely and laterally 3. Fibres travel upwards	1. Anterior arch of atlas 2. Transverse processes of fifth and sixth cervical vertebrae 3. Bodies of second, third and fourth cervical vertebrae	1. Forward-flexes cervical column, laterally rotates and laterally flexes neck 2. Commonly injured in 'whiplash' – cervical hyperextension injuries	C2–7

Table 1.3 Continued

Muscle	Origin	Route	Insertion	Action	Innervation
Longus capitis	Anterior tubercles of transverse processes of third to sixth cervical vertebrae	Fibres ascend, converging towards opposite side	Basilar part of occipital bone anterior to foramen magnum	Bilaterally, forward-flexes neck Unilaterally, laterally rotates neck	C1–3
Rectus capitis anterior	Anterior base of transverse process of the atlas	Fibres pass obliquely and medially upwards	Basilar part of occipital bone anterior to foramen magnum	Forward-flexes neck at atlanto-occipital junction	C2, C3
Rectus capitis lateralis	Transverse process of atlas	Fibres pass upwards	Jugular process of occipital bone	Laterally flexes neck at atlanto-occipital junction	C2, C3
Scalenus anterior	Anterior tubercles of transverse processes of third to sixth cervical vertebrae	Fibres descend almost vertically	Scalene tubercle (inner border of first rib)	Accessory muscle of respiration – raises first rib during inspiration Bilaterally, forward-flex neck Unilaterally, laterally flexes, rotates the neck	Ventral rami of cervical nn.

Table 1.3 Muscles of the neck (continued)

Muscle	Origin	Route	Insertion	Action	Innervation
Scalenus medius	Posterior tubercles of transverse processes of lower six cervical vertebrae	Fibres descend alongside vertebral column	Upper surface of first rib between scalene tubercle and subclavian groove	Accessory muscle of respiration – raises the first rib during inspiration Bilaterally, forward-flexes neck Unilaterally, laterally flexes, rotates the neck	Ventral rami of cervical nn.
Scalenus posterior	Posterior tubercles of transverse processes of lower two cervical vertebrae	Fibres descend laterally	Outer surface of second rib	Accessory muscle of respiration – raises the second rib during inspiration Bilaterally, forward-flexes neck Unilaterally, laterally flexes, rotates the neck	Ventral rami of lower cervical nn.

Table 1.3 Continued

Muscle	Origin	Route	Insertion	Action	Innervation
Rectus capitis posterior major	Spinous process of axis	Fibres pass upwards and laterally	Lateral part of inferior nuchal line of occipital bone	Extends and laterally rotates head	Suboccipital n.
Rectus capitis posterior minor	Tubercle on posterior arch of the atlas	Fibres pass upwards	Medial part of inferior nuchal line of occipital bone	Extends head	Suboccipital n.
Obliquus capitis inferior	Spinous process of axis	Fibres pass laterally and upwards	Transverse process of atlas	Laterally rotates atlas	Suboccipital n.
Obliquus capitis superior	Transverse process of atlas	Fibres pass posteriorly and superiorly	Occipital bone between superior and inferior nuchal line	Extends and laterally flexes head	Suboccipital n.

[a]Strap muscles.

Table 1.4 Intrinsic muscles of the larynx

Muscle	Origin	Course	Insertion	Action	Innervation
Oblique arytenoid	Posterior surface and lateral border of arytenoid cartilage	Fibres cross each other behind the arytenoid cartilages	Posterior surface of contralateral arytenoid cartilage near the apex	Adduct vocal folds by drawing arytenoid cartilages together	Inferior laryngeal branch of recurrent laryngeal branch of vagus n.
Aryepiglottic muscle	Apex of arytenoids cartilage	Fibres travel upwards	Epiglottis	Draws epiglottis posteriorly and downwards during swallowing	Inferior laryngeal branch of recurrent laryngeal branch of vagus n.
Transverse arytenoid	Posterior surface of arytenoid cartilage	Fibres pass horizontally	Posterior surface of contralateral arytenoid cartilage	Adduct vocal folds by drawing arytenoid cartilages together	Inferior laryngeal branch of recurrent laryngeal branch of vagus n.
Thyroepiglottic muscle	Inner surface of the thyroid cartilage near the laryngeal prominence	Fibres sweep upwards	Lateral surface of epiglottis	Draws epiglottis forwards, opening laryngeal inlet	Inferior laryngeal branch of recurrent laryngeal branch of vagus n.
Lateral cricoarytenoid	Lateral surface of cricoid cartilage	Fibres run obliquely	Muscular process of unilateral arytenoid cartilage	Draws muscular process of the arytenoid cartilage anteriorly, which pivots the arytenoid cartilage and adducts the vocal folds	Inferior laryngeal branch of recurrent laryngeal branch of vagus n.
Posterior cricoarytenoid	Posterior surface of lamina of cricoid cartilage	Fibres converge	Muscular process of unilateral arytenoid cartilage	Abduct vocal folds	Inferior laryngeal branch of recurrent laryngeal branch of vagus n.
Thyroarytenoid	Inner surface of thyroid cartilage	Fibres sweep backwards	Anterolateral surface of arytenoid cartilage	Draws the arytenoid cartilage forwards, relaxing and adducting the vocal folds	Inferior laryngeal branch of recurrent laryngeal branch of vagus n.
Cricothyroid	Arch of cricoid cartilage	Fibres travel forwards	Inferior cornu and lamina of thyroid cartilage	Draws the thyroid cartilage forwards, lengthening the vocal ligaments	External branch of superior laryngeal branch of vagus n.
Vocalis	Surface of the thyroid cartilage, vocal process of the arytenoid cartilage	Fibres form a triangular band	Vocal ligament	Adjusts pitch by relaxing segments of the vocal ligament	Inferior laryngeal branch of recurrent laryngeal branch of vagus n.

Table 1.5 Intrinsic muscles of the pharynx

Muscle	Origin	Course	Insertion	Action	Innervation
Middle constrictor	Greater horn of the hyoid bone, inferior part of the stylohyoid ligament	Fibres sweep round to the back of the pharynx outside lowermost fibres of superior constrictor	Midline pharyngeal raphe	Constricts pharynx	Vagus n.
Inferior constrictor	Oblique line of the thyroid cartilage, lateral surface of cricoid cartilage	Fibres sweep round to the back of the pharynx outside lowermost fibres of middle constrictor	Midline pharyngeal raphe	Constricts pharynx	Vagus n., via the pharyngeal plexus, with aid from the superior laryngeal and recurrent laryngeal nerves
Tensor palati	Scaphoid fossa, lateral wall of the auditory tube cartilage	Fibres run down the outside of the superior constrictor and converge to a delicate tendon, looping round the pterygoid humulus	Palatine aponeurosis	Opens the auditory tube, tenses the soft palate	Mandibular branch of trigeminal n.
Levator palati	Apex of petrous part of temporal bone and medial surface of the auditory tube cartilage	Fibres run over the top of the superior constrictor	Muscles and fascia of the soft palate, palatine aponeurosis	Elevates the soft palate	Vagus n.
Styloglossus	Anterior and lateral surfaces of styloid process	Fibres pass downwards and forwards between internal and external carotid arteries	Posterolateral side of the tongue	Draws up sides of the tongue, retracts the tongue	Hypoglossal n.
Hyoglossus	Body of hyoid bone and upper border of greater horn of hyoid	Fibres pass almost vertically upwards	Side of the tongue	Depresses sides of the tongue, retracts tongue	Hypoglossal n.

Table 1.5 Intrinsic muscles of the pharynx (continued)

Muscle	Origin	Course	Insertion	Action	Innervation
Genioglossus	Mental spine of mandible	Fibres fan out	Dorsum of tongue, body of hyoid	Inferior fibres protrude the tongue, middle fibres depress the tongue, superior fibres draw the tip back and down	Hypoglossal n.
Palatoglossus	Palatine aponeurosis	Fibres are continuous with the muscle of the opposite side, passing downwards, forwards and laterally in front of the palatine tonsil	Side of the tongue	Elevates and retracts the tongue	Vagus n.
Salpingopharyngeus	Inferior surface of the anteromedial end of the auditory tube cartilage	Fibres travel downwards	Pharyngeal wall and superior border of the thyroid cartilage along with palatopharyngeus m.	Raises the nasopharynx during deglutition and laterally draws the pharyngeal walls up	Vagus n.
Palatopharyngeus	Posterior margin of hard palate and palatine aponeurosis	Fibres pass downwards and laterally behind the palatine tonsil	Posterior margin of thyroid cartilage, posterior wall of the pharynx	Elevates larynx and pharynx	Vagus n.
Stylopharyngeus	Medial side of styloid process	Fibres pass downwards along the side of the pharynx between the superior constrictor and the middle constrictor	Superior border of thyroid cartilage and pharyngeal wall	Elevates the pharynx, elevates the larynx, aids swallowing by dilating pharynx	Glossopharyngeal n.

Table 1.6 Arteries of the neck

Artery	Origin	Relations	Termination	Branches
Common carotid a.	On the right from the bifurcation of the brachiocephalic trunk behind the sternoclavicular joint. On the left from the aortic arch	**Superficial** Sternomastoid artery from the superior thyroid a. CN XII Ansa hypoglossi Internal jugular v. Anterior jugular v. Middle thyroid v. Sternocleidomastoid Sternohyoid Sternothyroid Omohyoid **Deep** Thoracic duct Subclavian a. Vertebral a. Inferior thyroid a. Sympathetic trunk Middle cervical ganglion CN X Recurrent laryngeal nn. Longus cervicis Longus capitis	By dividing into external and internal carotids at upper border of thyroid cartilage opposite C4	Bifurcates into internal and external carotid aa.

Table 1.6 Arteries of the neck (continued)

Artery	Origin	Relations	Termination	Branches
(Common carotid a.)		**Medial** Larynx Trachea Pharynx Oesophagus Recurrent laryngeal nn. Thyroid body **Lateral** Internal jugular v. CN X Apex of lung and pleura		
External carotid a.	Bifurcation of common carotid at upper border of thyroid cartilage opposite C4	**Superficial** The parotid gland that envelopes the artery Styloid process CN VII, XII Sternocleidomastoid Posterior belly of digastric Stylohyoid Superior thyroid v. Lingual v. Common facial v. Posterior facial v.	Opposite the neck of the condyle of the mandible by subdivision into superficial temporal and maxillary arteries	(*Mnemonic*: **S**ome **A**natomists **L**ike **F**reaking **O**ut **P**oor **M**edical **S**tudents) **S**uperior thyroid **A**scending pharyngeal **L**ingual **F**acial **O**ccipital **P**osterior auricular **M**axillary **S**uperficial temporal

Table 1.6 Continued

Artery	Origin	Relations	Termination	Branches
		Deep Ascending pharyngeal a. Internal carotid a. CN IX Pharyngeal branch of vagus Internal laryngeal n. External laryngeal n. Styloglossus Stylopharyngeus Constrictors of pharynx		
Superior thyroid a.	From external carotid close to its origin	–	By distribution to the anterior surface of thyroid body in its proximal two-thirds	Muscular Infrahyoid Superior laryngeal Sternomastoid Cricothyroid Glandular (thyroid)

Table 1.6 Arteries of the neck (continued)

Artery	Origin	Relations	Termination	Branches
Lingual a.	From the external carotid opposite the tip of the greater cornu of the hyoid bone	**Superficial** Submandibular duct CN XII Lingual n. Digastric Stylohyoid Hyoglossus Mylohyoid **Deep** Middle constrictor Stylohyoid ligament Genioglossus	As profunda linguae to tip of the tongue	Suprahyoid Dorsalis linguae Sublingual
Facial a.	From external carotid 1.25 cm above the tip of the greater cornu of the hyoid	–	At the medial canthus	Ascending palatine Tonsillar Glandular Submental Inferior labial Superior labial Lateral nasal Muscular

Table 1.6 Continued

Artery	Origin	Relations	Termination	Branches
Maxillary a.	Opposite and deep to the neck of the condyle of the mandible from the bifurcation of the external carotid. It passes deeply to the mandible in its course		In the pterygopalatine fossa by subdivision into its terminal branches	Course is divided into three parts by the lateral pterygoid m. **First part proximal to lateral pterygoid:** Deep auricular Anterior tympanic Middle meningeal Accessory meningeal Inferior alveolar and mylohyoid br. **Second part superficial to lateral pterygoid:** Deep temporal Pterygoid Masseteric Buccal

Table 1.6 Arteries of the neck (continued)

Artery	Origin	Relations	Termination	Branches
(Maxillary a.)				**Third part in the pterygopalatine fossa:** Posterior superior alveolar Infraorbital and superior alveolar br. Artery of the pterygoid canal Palatine branches including descending to greater and lesser palatine Pharyngeal Sphenopalatine (anastomosis with greater palatine)

Table 1.6 Continued

Artery	Origin	Relations	Termination	Branches
Internal carotid a.	From the bifurcation of the common carotid at the upper border of the thyroid cartilage opposite C4		At the anterior perforated substance, subdividing into anterior and middle cerebrals	Caroticotympanic Pterygoid Cavernous Dural Pituitary Ganglionic (trigeminal ganglion) Ophthalmic Posterior communicating Choroidal Anterior cerebral Middle cerebral
Ophthalmic a.	From the internal carotid after perforation of the dura on the medial side of anterior clinoid process		At the anterior part of the orbit by subdivision into dorsal nasal and supratrochlear aa.	Lacrimal Supraorbital Meningeal Retinal Ciliary Anterior and posterior ethmoidal Medial palpebral Supratrochlear Dorsal nasal

Table 1.6 Arteries of the neck (continued)

Artery	Origin	Relations	Termination	Branches
Vertebral a.	First part of subclavian artery	Reaches the transversarium foramen of the sixth cervical vertebra through the other foramina. Exiting from the first transversarium it passes medially from the foramen transversarium of the atlas to pierce the posterior atlanto-occipital membrane. Here it has a sinuous course. It enters the cranial cavity through the foramen magnum to the anterior aspect of the brain stem	As the basilar artery in the cranial cavity	**Basilar:** Cerebellar Pontine Posterior cerebral **Anterior spinal**
Thyrocervical trunk	First part of the subclavian a.	At the medial border of the scalenus anterior muscle	Terminal branches after a short course	Inferior thyroid Suprascapular Transverse cervical
Costocervical trunk	Second part of subclavian a.	Posterior to scalenus anterior muscle	Into terminal branches	Highest intercostal artery Deep cervical

Table 1.7 Head and neck veins

Vein	Origin	Relations	Termination	Tributaries
Internal jugular v.	At the jugular foramen as the continuation of the sigmoid sinus	Runs within the carotid sheath	At the sternoclavicular joint by joining the subclavian to form the brachiocephalic vein	Common facial Thyroid Lingual Inferior petrosal sinus Pharyngeal
External jugular v.	Posterior branch of retromandibular vein and posterior auricular vein	Runs superficial to the sternocleidomastoid in the superficial fascia of the neck from the earlobe to the midclavicle	Subclavian v.	Superficial temporal Transverse facial Maxillary Retromandibular Posterior auricular
Anterior jugular v.	Midline of neck	Originally superficially, turns laterally deep to the sternocleidomastoid	Internal jugular or subclavian vv.	Submandibular region Anterior venous arch
Retromandibular v.	Confluence of superficial temporal and maxillary vv.	Superficially posterior to the angle of the mandible it divides into anterior and posterior branches. Anterior branch joins the facial vein. Posterior branch joins the posterior auricular vein forming the external jugular	See Relations	Superficial temporal Maxillary
Facial v.	Angular v. (confluence of supraorbital and supratrochlear vv.)	Runs with facial a. to border of mandible	Joins retromandibular v. after piercing deep investing fascia at mandible	Supraorbital Supratrochlear

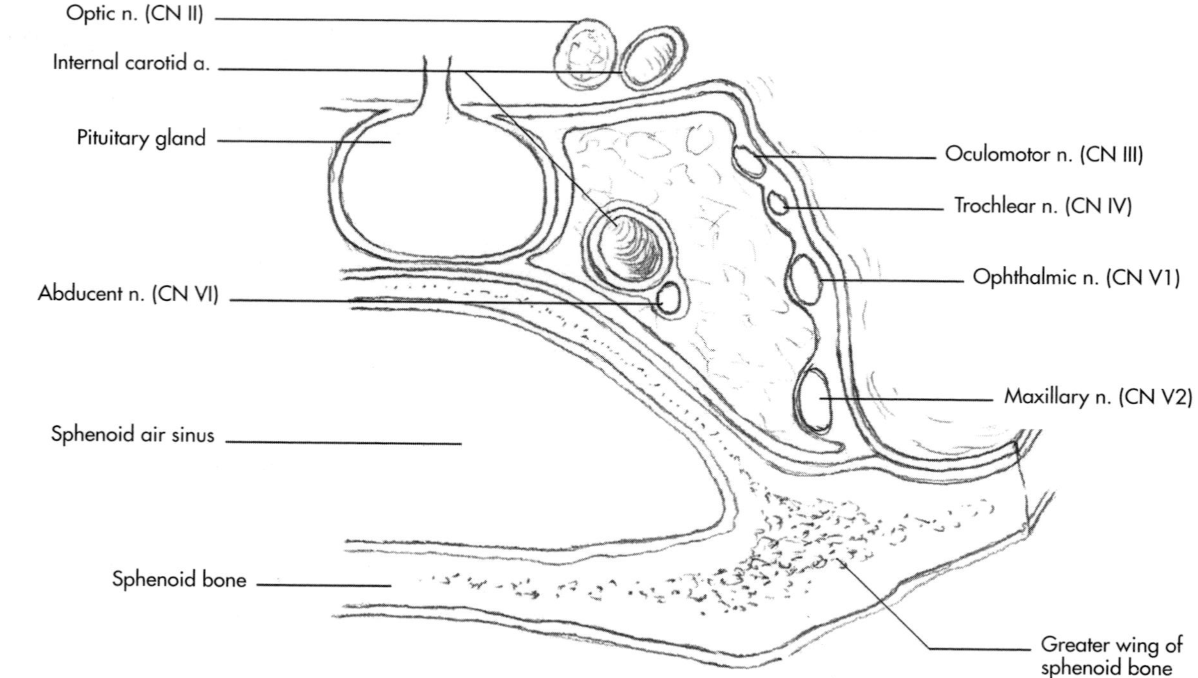

Figure 1.1 Cavernous sinus

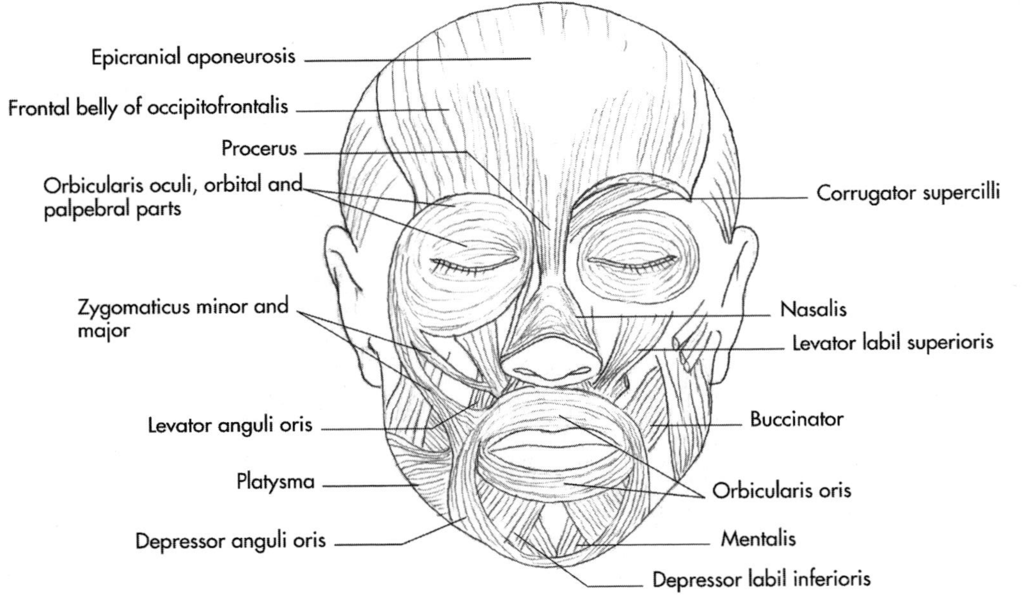

Figure 1.2 Muscles of facial expression

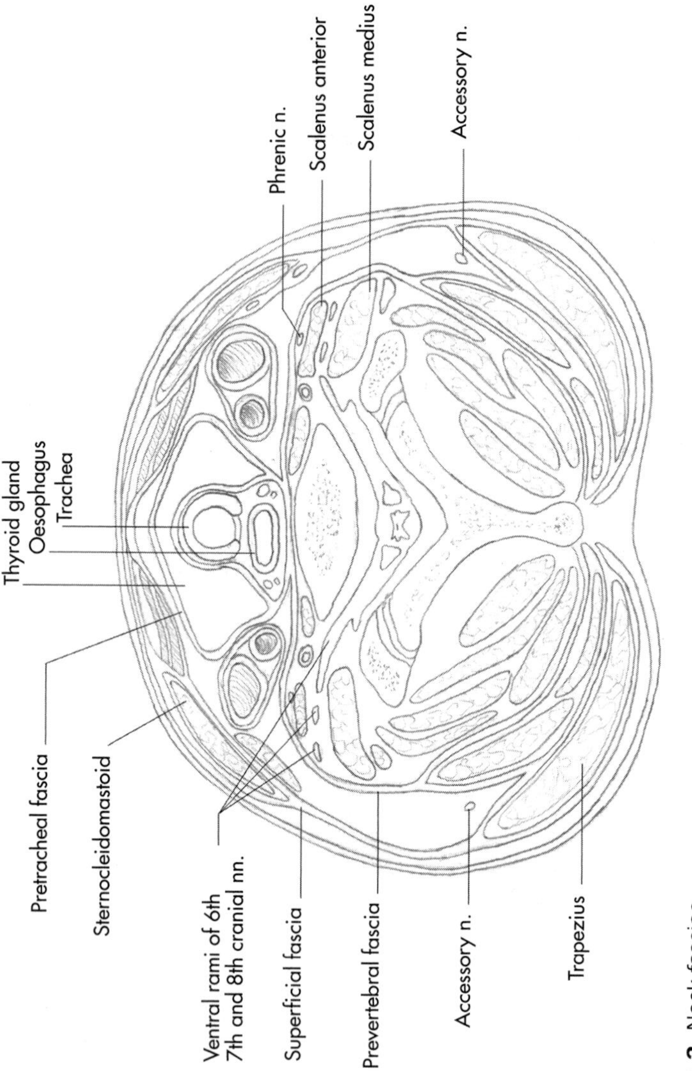

Thyroid gland
Oesophagus
Trachea
Phrenic n.
Scalenus anterior
Scalenus medius
Accessory n.
Pretracheal fascia
Sternocleidomastoid
Ventral rami of 6th 7th and 8th cranial nn.
Superficial fascia
Prevertebral fascia
Accessory n.
Trapezius

Figure 1.3 Neck fasciae

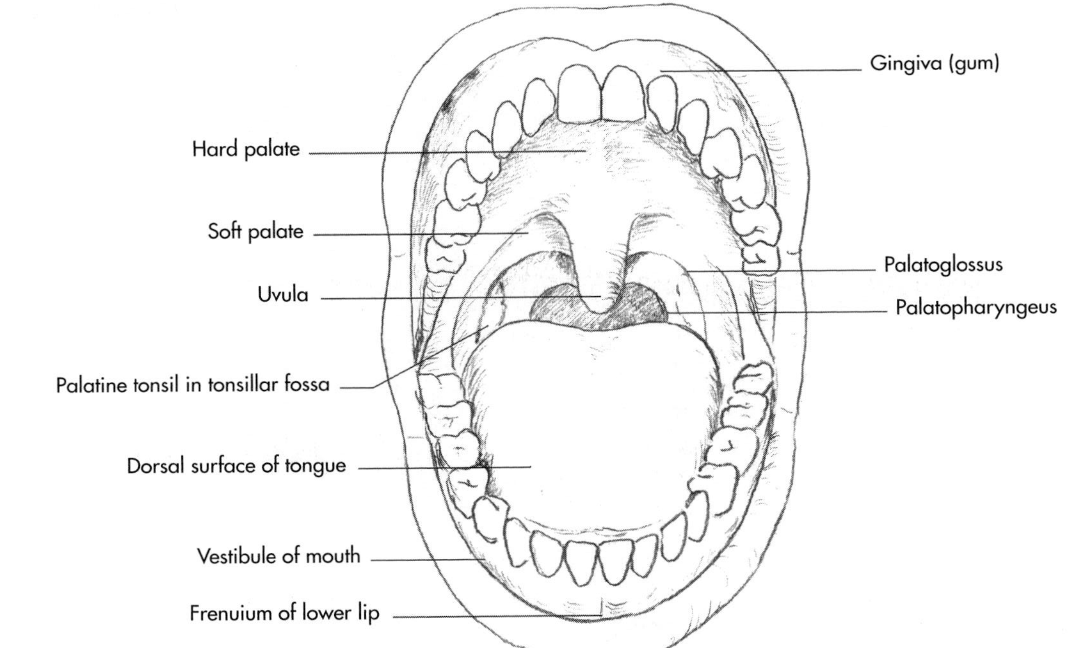

Figure 1.4 Oral cavity

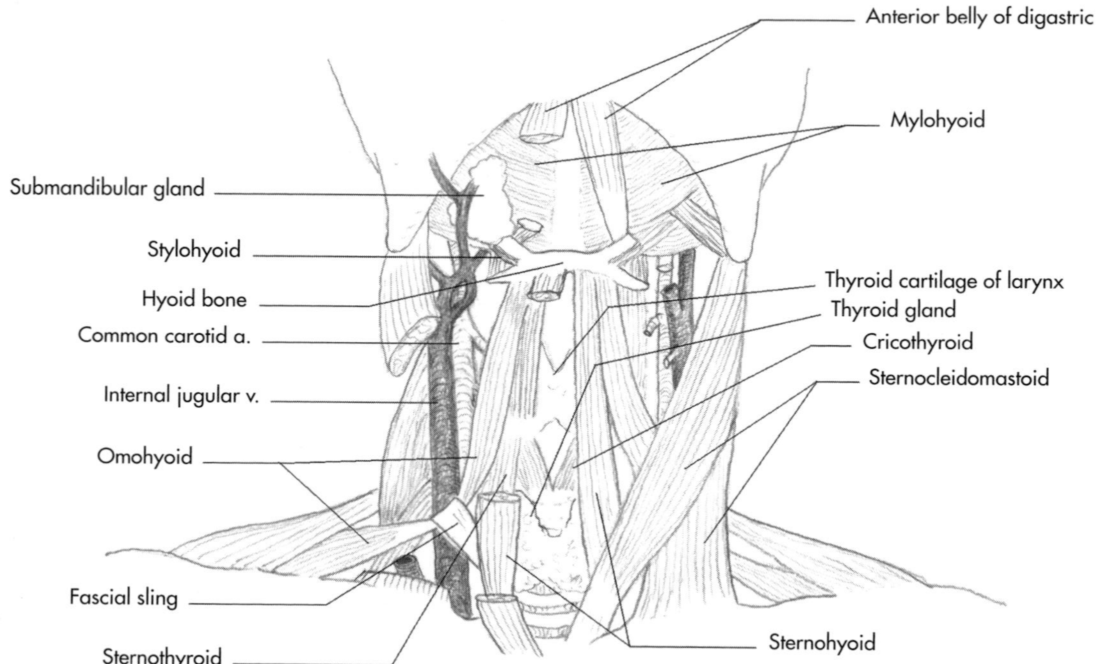

Figure 1.5 Anterior muscles of the neck

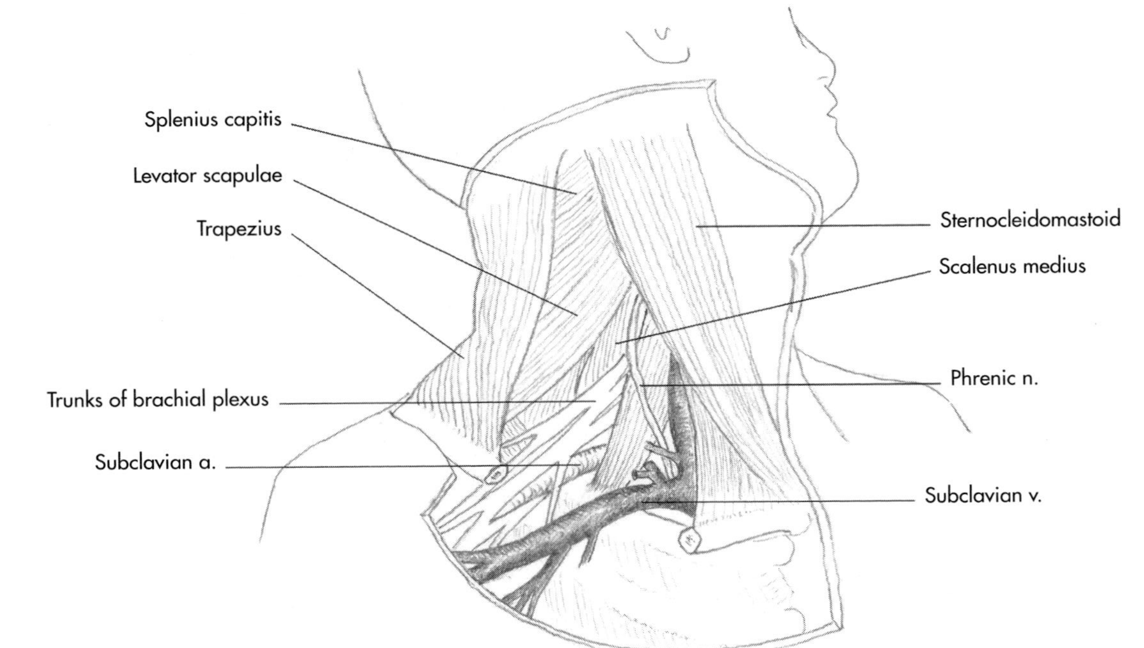

Figure 1.6 Deep dissection of the right posterior triangle of the neck

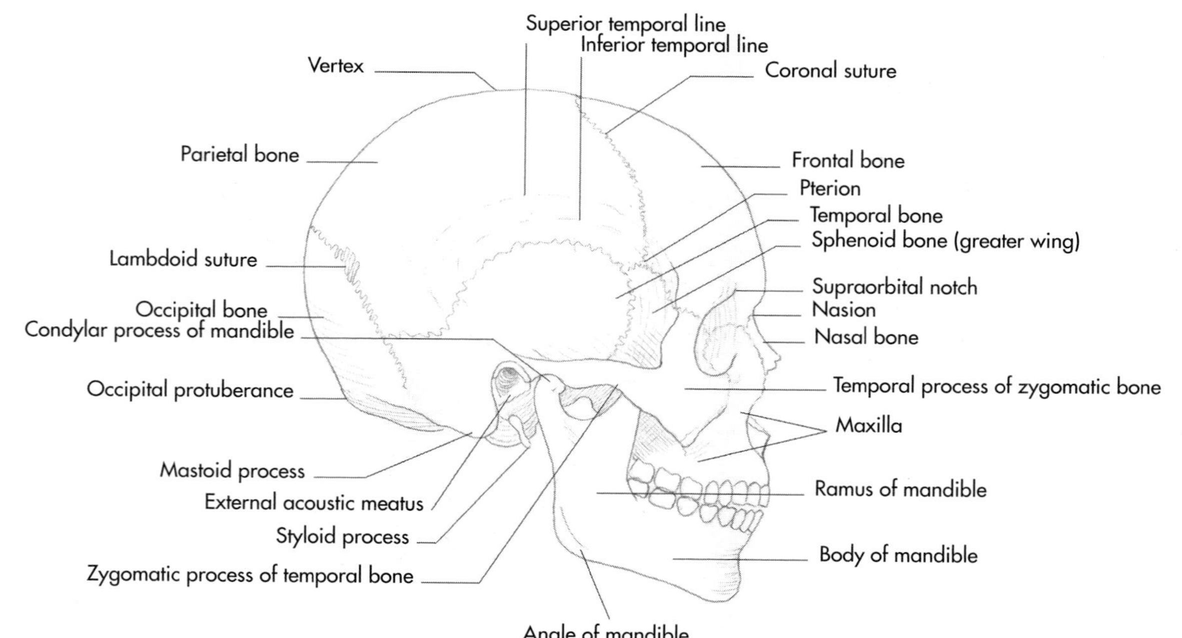

Figure 1.7 Skull

CHAPTER 2: THORAX

MEDIASTINUM

What is the mediastinum? The virtual space between the pleurae in the thoracic cavity.

What are its borders? Superiorly, the thoracic inlet; laterally, both pleurae; inferiorly, the diaphragm; anteriorly, the sternum; and, posteriorly, the thoracic vertebrae 1–12 (Figure 2.1).

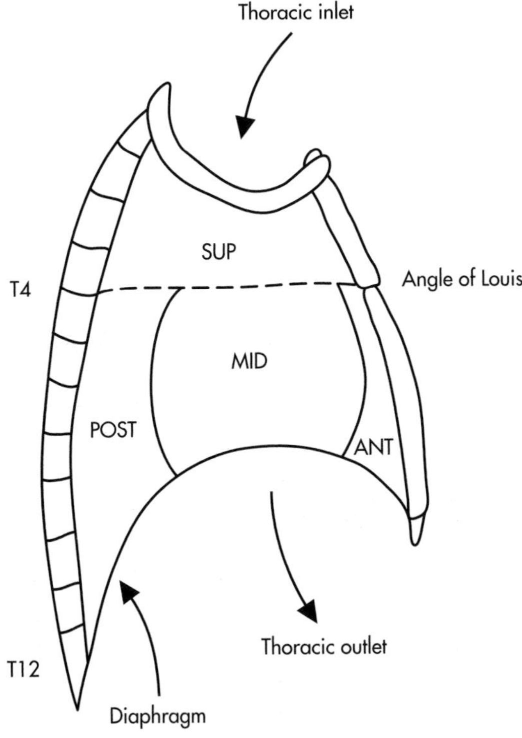

Figure 2.1

What are its divisions?

Superior and inferior mediastinum, divided by an imaginary transverse line from the manubriosternal junction anteriorly (angle of Louis) and T4 posteriorly. The superior mediastinum has no divisions but the inferior mediastinum is further divided into the anterior, middle and posterior mediastinum.

What are the contents of the superior mediastinum?

1. Thyroid gland.
2. Aortic arch and great vessels.
3. Oesophagus.
4. Trachea.
5. Vagus, recurrent laryngeal and phrenic nerves.

And of the anterior mediastinum?

1. Thymus gland.
2. Lymph nodes.
3. Internal mammary artery and vein.
4. Fat and connective tissue.

And of the middle mediastinum?

1. Heart.
2. Pulmonary arteries and veins.
3. Superior vena cava (SVC) and inferior vena cava (IVC).

And of the posterior mediastinum?

1. Oesophagus.
2. Descending thoracic aorta.
3. Azygos and hemiazygos veins.
4. Vagus and recurrent laryngeal nerves.

What are the surface markings of the diaphragm?

Fourth intercostal space on the right and fifth intercostal space on the left.

What is the blood supply of the diaphragm?

Pericardiophrenic and musculophrenic branches of the internal thoracic artery. Superior and inferior phrenic arteries and the intercostal artery.

What is the nerve supply and why is it important?

Phrenic nerve supplies the motor fibres. Sensory fibres run in the phrenic and lower intercostal nerves.

The phrenic nerve, originating mostly from C4 (also C3 and C5), is liable to paralysis in spinal cord injury above this level. Referred pain caused by an irritating abscess (e.g. subphrenic) is sensed in the C4 (shoulder) distribution as a result of simultaneous synapses on the same axons supplied by C4 afferent nerves. (*Mnemonic:* C3, 4 and 5 keep the diaphragm alive.)

What goes through the diaphragmatic apertures?

There are three diaphragmatic apertures:
1. The caval opening (at T8): the IVC and phrenic nerve.
2. The oesophageal hiatus (at T10): the oesophagus and vagal trunks.
3. The aortic hiatus (at T12): the descending thoracic aorta (becomes the abdominal aorta thereafter), azygos vein and thoracic duct.

How can the spinal levels of each aperture be remembered?

(*Mnemonic:* count the letters!)
Aortic hiatus = 12 letters = T12.
Oesophagus = 10 letters = T10.
Vena cava = 8 letters = T8.

HEART

What are the layers of the pericardium?

There is an outer fibrous pericardium that is fused with the central tendon of the diaphragm. The two parietal and visceral layers of serous pericardium in this potential space can fill with fluid (inflammation) or blood, constricting cardiac pumping ability. A needle might have to be introduced between the xiphisternum and the costal cartilage for aspiration.

What is the blood supply of the heart?

The right and left coronary arteries originate from the ascending aortic sinus. The left coronary artery (LCA) from the left posterior aortic sinus and the right coronary artery (RCA) from the anterior aortic sinus.

What does the LCA supply?

This is larger in calibre than the RCA and supplies the majority of the left atrium and ventricle as well as the interventricular septum.

What are the branches of the LCA?

The left main stem continues as the left anterior descending artery but also gives branches to the diagonal and circumflex arteries.

What does the RCA supply?

The right atrium and ventricle.

What are the branches of the RCA?

Right posterior descending artery (in 30% of people) and the marginal branches.

What does the term 'dominance' mean?

It describes the origin of the posterior descending artery where left dominance implies that the origin is the LCA (occurs in 70% of the population).

When does coronary blood flow take place?

During diastole, from the sinuses of Valsalva.

What is the venous drainage of the heart?

These mostly drain via small veins into the right atrium. A small amount drains directly into the right ventricle.

Where are the atrioventricular valves?

The mitral (bicuspid) valve separates the left atrium and left ventricle, and the tricuspid valve separates the right chambers. They are supported by the chordae tendinae.

Why are diseases more common on the left than right valves?

The left side of the heart houses the mitral and aortic valves, which are under high pressure to maintain the systemic circulation. The tricuspid and pulmonary valves serve the pulmonary circulation under low pressures.

Which arteries are used in a heart bypass operation?

The left internal thoracic artery is anastomosed to the anterior descending artery. The right internal thoracic is anastomosed either to the aorta or to the RCA.

How does the heart's conducting system work?

The sinoatrial node (pacemaker) lies in the upper right atrium, partially surrounding the SVC. The atrioventricular node lies in the interarterial septum close to the opening of the coronary sinus. The atrioventricular bundle travels to the muscular interventricular septum, as the bundle of His, where it divides into the left and right crura (branches). The moderator band carries the right branch to the right ventricle.

Where are the heart sounds heard?

Pulmonary: left side of sternal edge, second intercostal space.
Aortic: right side of sternal edge, second intercostal space.
Tricuspid: right side of sternal edge, fifth intercostal space.
Mitral: left midclavicular line, fifth intercostal space.

RESPIRATORY TREE

At what point does the trachea divide?

It divides into the right and left main bronchi at the level of T3–4. This is known as the carina.

Where are foreign bodies most likely to lodge?

The right lower lobe, for three reasons:
1. The right main bronchus has a wider lumen than the left main

bronchus because it delivers air to the bigger lung.
2. The left main bronchus has a more acute angle than the left after bifurcation because it lies under the arch of the aorta.
3. The carina lies slightly to the left.

What are the bronchial divisions?

The main (primary) bronchi divide into the lobar (secondary) bronchi, which further subdivide into the segmental (tertiary) bronchi. These supply the bronchopulmonary segments in each lung.

What are the bronchial divisions of each lung?

The right lung: three lobes – the superior, middle and inferior. These are further subdivided into ten bronchopulmonary segments.
The left lung: two lobes – the superior and inferior. The lingual is the remnant of the left middle lobe found at the lower aspect of the left upper lobe. There are eight to ten bronchopulmonary segments.

What is the surface anatomy of the lungs?

The pleural cavities extend to the twelfth rib posteriorly and to the eighth rib anteriorly. The lungs extend to the tenth rib posteriorly and to the sixth rib anteriorly. Both the lung and the pleural cavity lie above the level of the thoracic cavity superiorly, so exposing it to injury.

Why is the costodiaphragmatic recess important clinically?

It is this region where lung signs are picked up clinically. Dullness and reduced breath sounds occur here in pulmonary effusions.

What is the blood supply to lungs?

Small bronchial arteries supply the tissue of the lungs, the bronchial tree and the pulmonary pleura. The two left bronchial arteries arise directly

	from the aorta. The single right bronchial artery arises from the third right posterior intercostal artery. The veins drain into the azygos or pulmonary veins.
Where do vessels and bronchi enter the lung?	At the hilum.
How many layers of pleura are there?	Two: the outer parietal layer is attached to the chest wall and the inner visceral layer is attached to the lungs. The parietal pleura around the mediastinum is known as the mediastinal pleura.
What is pleural fluid?	A serous lining secreted by the pleural mesothelium into the potential space between the two layers of pleura. It allows lubrication during respiration.

THORACIC WALL

What is the most commonly fractured bone in the body?	The clavicle.
What is the weakest point of the clavicle?	The junction between the middle and lateral thirds.
What are the relations of the clavicle?	Behind the medial third: subclavian vessels trunks of the brachial plexus. Behind the sternoclavicular joint: left common carotid artery (on the left) and the bifurcation of the brachiocephalic artery (on the right). The internal jugular vein lateral to the previously mentioned arteries.
What is Virchow's node/Troissier's sign?	The presence of a palpable Virchow's node in the supraclavicular fossa on the left side is a positive Troissier's

sign. The node is classically palpated in metastatic gastric cancer.

What is found in the intercostal space?

Superficial to deep: external inner and innermost muscles. The neurovascular bundle lies between the inner (internal oblique) and innermost (subcostal and transversus thoracis) intercostal muscles. The vein lies superiorly; then the artery, followed by the nerve inferiorly, lies below the costal groove, exposing it for infiltration with local anaesthetic.

How can this be remembered?

(*Mnemonic:* **VAN** [superiorly to inferiorly].)
Vein.
Artery.
Nerve.

How do you drain pleuritic fluid?

Insertion of a wide-bore needle at the upper border of the lower rib so as not to damage the neurovascular bundle. Local anaesthetic is infiltrated superficially into the skin first.

BREAST

What is the breast made up of?

Ten to 20 lobes containing connective tissue, fat, glandular tissue and the duct system. There is a single lactiferous duct from each lobe opening at the nipple.

What is Cooper's ligament?

Fibrous bands that divide the breast parenchyma into 12–20 separate lobules of glandular tissue and suspend the breast by superior attachments.

What is the arterial supply of the breast?

The pectoral branch of the thoracoacromial artery anastomoses with the internal mammary artery and the external mammary branch of the lateral thoracic artery to supply the breast. Perforating thoracic branches of the intercostals also contribute. A subdermal plexus supplies the skin.

What is the venous drainage of the breast?

The circulus venosus is an anastomotic circle around the base of the nipple. Veins branch out radially from here and drain into the axillary and internal mammary veins.

What is the lymphatic drainage of the breast?

Medially: parasternal.
Axillary: (75%) pectoral, subcostal, central, apical (from level I to level III in axillary clearance).
Superior: supraclavicular and infraclavicular.

How is the breast innervated?

With lots of overlap. Anterior and lateral branches of the fourth, fifth and sixth intercostal nerves provide innervation in a dermatomal fashion. The nipple lies in the dermatome of the fourth intercostal nerve, which has a deep and a superficial branch. The **deep branch** passes inferolaterally on the pectoralis major fascia then courses up to supply the areola. The **superficial branch** passes up through the superficial parenchyma.

What are the relations of the breast?

The breast lies within the superficial fascia with the second rib above and the sixth rib below. It extends medially from the lateral border of the sternum to the midaxillary line laterally.
The **axillary tail** of the breast extends up into the base of the axilla.
The breast is separated from pectoralis major and its investing fascia by a layer of loose connective tissue.

AXILLA

What is the axilla?

The axilla, or armpit, is a pyramidal region of the body between the arm and thorax. It provides a passageway for the important large arteries, nerves, veins and lymphatics. It has an apex and floor, and anterior, posterior, lateral and medial walls.

What are the boundaries of the axilla?

Apex: convergence of the clavicle (anterior), the scapula (posterior) and the first rib (medially).
Floor: formed by the skin and fascia of the concave axilla (armpit).
Anterior wall: pectoralis major covering pectoralis minor and subclavius.
Posterior wall: subscapularis, latissimus dorsi and teres major (from above downwards).
Lateral wall: long head of biceps and coracobrachialis (in the bicipital groove).
Medial wall: serratus anterior (covering upper four ribs).

What are the contents of the axilla?

Axillary artery and its branches.
Axillary vein and its tributaries.
Intercostobrachial nerve.
Brachial plexus.
Axillary lymph nodes.
Fat.

What drains to the axillary lymph nodes?

Lymph from the upper limb, shoulder and scapular regions, pectoral region (including the mammary gland) and upper abdomen drains into the axillary nodes.

What are the groups of lymph nodes found in the axilla?

Pectoral (anterior), subscapular (posterior), lateral, central and apical.

How many nodes are there? 15–20 nodes.

What is the distribution and drainage of these nodes? See table 2.1.

Table 2.1

Group	Location	Afferents (regions drained)	Efferents to	Notes
Pectoral (anterior)	Along the lateral border of the pectoralis major m.	From the lateral part of the breast and anterolateral thoracic and abdominal wall to the level of the umbilicus	Central nodes	Level 1
Subscapular (posterior)	Along the subscapular vessels	From the back down to the umbilicus and back of the neck	Central nodes	Level 1
Lateral	Along the distal axillary v.	From the upper limb	Central nodes	Level 1
Central	In the fat of the axilla	From pectoral, subscapular and lateral lymph nodes	Apical nodes	Level 2
Apical	Apex of the axilla	From all axillary lymph nodes	Subclavian trunk	Level 3

Why are the axillary nodes important clinically? Axillary lymph node levels are of special importance in breast cancer spread and dissection. They are grouped into three levels according to their relation to the pectoralis minor muscle:

Level 1: lateral to pectoralis minor muscle.
Level 2: posterior to it.
Level 3: medial to it.

OESOPHAGUS

What is the oesophagus?	A muscular tube extending from the cricoid cartilage (C6) to the gastro-oesophageal junction (T10).
What is the distance from the top incisor teeth to the gastro-oesophageal junction?	40 cm.
How long is the oesophagus?	25 cm.
What is it lined with?	Stratified squamous epithelium.
What type of muscle is it made of?	Depends on the level: **upper third:** striated. **middle third:** striated and smooth. **lower third:** smooth. The muscles themselves are arranged as an outer, longitudinal layer and an inner, circular layer.
What are its narrowest points?	There are three (distances given are measured from the front incisor teeth): 1. Cricopharyngeal sphincter (15 cm). 2. At the aortic arch (22 cm). 3. Where it crosses the diaphragm (38 cm).
How much of the oesophagus is intra-abdominal?	2 cm.
What are the branches of the abdominal aorta from superior to inferior?	**Unpaired:** 1. Coeliac trunk 2. Superior mesenteric artery 3. Inferior mesenteric artery 4. Median sacral artery (at bifurcation). **Paired (visceral):** 1. Adrenal arteries 2. Renal arteries

3. Gonadal arteries (ovarian/testicular).

Paired (abdominal wall):

1. Subcostal arteries
2. Inferior phrenic arteries.
3. Lumbar arteries (five on each side).

Table 2.2 Thoracic muscles

Muscle	Origin	Insertion	Action	Innervation
External intercostal	Lower border of rib	Upper border of rib Deficient anteriorly, replaced with fibrous membrane	Runs forwards Elevates thoracic cavity in AP axis Increases transverse thoracic diameter	Intercostal n.
Internal intercostal	Lower border of rib	Upper border of rib Deep to external intercostal	Runs backwards Elevates thoracic cavity in AP axis Increases transverse thoracic diameter	Intercostal n.
Innermost intercostal (subcostal) (transversus thoracis)	Deep surface of rib	Discontinuous to deep surface of ribs, costal cartilage and sternum	Runs forwards Elevates thoracic cavity in AP axis Increases transverse thoracic diameter	Intercostal n.
Diaphragm	Inner aspect of thoracic outlet Xiphisternum Lower six ribs Costal cartilages		Increases size of thoracic cavity via a negative pressure system	Phrenic n.

AP, anteroposterior.

Table 2.3 Thoracic nerves

Nerve	Source	Course and relations	Branches	Type
Thoracic sympathetic trunk (sympathetic outflow for the body)	Spinal cord preganglionic nerves (T1–L2). Synapse within the sympathetic trunk ganglia	Extend from the base of skull to coccyx. There are 3 cervical, 11 thoracic, 4 lumbar and 4 sacral ganglia within the length of the trunk. The trunk contains preganglionic sympathetic nerves. The first thoracic ganglion is fused with the inferior cervical ganglion to form the stellate ganglion. Paravertebral course on the heads of the ribs posteriorly, coming to lie distally on the bodies of the vertebrae. The two trunks pass behind the medial arcuate ligament on the surface of the psoas m. Each sympathetic ganglion is associated with an intercostal space	Supply thorax, head and neck sympathetic innervation **Abdomen:** Greater splanchnic nn. (T5–9 ganglia) (5) Lesser splanchnic nn. (T9–11 ganglia) (4) Least splanchnic nn. (T12–L2 ganglia) (3)	**Sensory:** Thoracic autonomic plexus: cardiac, pulmonary, oesophageal, abdominal autonomic plexus
Intercostal nerves T1–12 (thoracic spinal nn.)	Spinal cord	Upper border of space, below rib in costal groove	T1 contributes to brachial plexus to the upper limb T7–11 travel beneath costal margin of the rib T12 (subcostal n): runs below 12th rib Intercostobrachial n. Lateral cutaneous branch Collateral br. (lower border of space) Anterior cutaneous br. (skin over the midline)	**Motor:** Intercostals Abdominal wall **Sensory:** Lateral + anterior thoracic and abdominal wall

Table 2.3 Thoracic nerves (continued)

Nerve	Source	Course and relations	Branches	Type
Intercostobrachial n.	Lateral cutaneous br. of T2	Through the axilla. Serratus anterior m. lies medially in the axilla	–	**Sensory:** Medial surface of upper arm
Subcostal n.	Spinal cord (T12)	Lower aspect of 12th rib. Emerges posteriorly to lateral arcuate ligament of diaphragm lying on quadratus laborum and penetrating transversus abdominis to enter neurovascular plane posterior to the upper kidney on the posterior abdominal wall	–	**Motor:** Lower rectus abdominis **Sensory:** Skin of T12 dermatome
Phrenic n.	Ventral rami: C3, 4, 5 (keeps the diaphragm alive!)	Lies on the anterior surface of scalenus anterior. Enters thoracic cavity over first rib medial to scalenus anterior Both are also joined by the cardiophrenic arteries as they reach the pericardium **Right:** lateral to internal jugular, passing posterior to the R. subclavian v. and lateral to R. brachiocephalic and SVC, on to pericardium anterior to the hilum **Left:** descending lateral to L. subclavian a., is deep to L. brachiocephalic v. It crosses anterior to the arch of the aorta and L. pulmonary a. on to the pericardium anterior to the hilum towards the diaphragm	Diaphragmatic Pleural Pericardial Inferior vena caval Peritoneal: hepatic, adrenal	**Motor:** Diaphragm **Sensory:** Mediastinum Pericardium Diaphragm Pericardium Peritoneum

Table 2.3 Continued

Nerve	Source	Course and relations	Branches	Type
Vagus n. (CN X)	Dorsal motor nucleus of vagus (visceral motor), nucleus ambiguus (branchial motor), nucleus solitarius (taste and visceral sensory) and sensory nucleus of trigeminal n. (common sensation with trigeminal n.)	**Right:** behind and medial to R. brachiocephalic v. It courses towards the left, with the L. brachiocephalic passing anteriorly, towards the trachea. It gives off the R. recurrent branch here and continues posterior to the hilum and on to the oesophagus **Left:** between the L. common carotid and L. subclavian arteries deep to the brachiocephalic v., over the arch of the aorta, following it distally. It is then posterior to the L. pulmonary a., posterior to the hilum	L. + R. recurrent laryngeal n. Pulmonary (anterior + posterior) Oesophageal plexus (anterior + posterior) continuing as anterior + posterior vagal trunks with the oesophagus into the abdomen	**Motor:** Larynx (recurrent laryngeal) **Sensory:** Thoracic viscera plexus (parasympathetic stimulation)

Table 2.4 Thoracic arteries

Artery	Origin	Relations	Termination	Branches	Supply
Posterior intercostal aa.	Aorta Upper two intercostal aa. derived from supreme intercostal a. from costocervical trunk	Intercostal nerves and veins Costal grooves	Anastomosis with anterior intercostal aa. from internal thoracic	Dorsal branches Spinal branches	Vertebral bodies, meninges and spinal cord
Internal thoracic (internal mammary) a.	Branch of first part of subclavian in root of neck at the medial edge of scalenus anterior	**Anterior:** descends in the thorax deep to the cartilages of the upper six ribs just lateral to the sternum **Posterior:** pericardium, heart and transversus thoracis m.	Sixth intercostal space by subdivision into superior epigastric and musculophrenic aa.	Sixth anterior intercostal aa. Pericardiophrenic a. Superior epigastric a. Musculophrenic a.	Rib cage, pericardium, diaphragm, anterior abdominal wall mm.
Musculophrenic a.	Internal thoracic a.	Continues around costal margin	Terminal branches to diaphragm	Anterior intercostal aa.	Diaphragm
Superior epigastric a.	Internal thoracic (sixth intercostal space)	Enters abdomen between the sternum and diaphragm	Anastomosis with inferior epigastic a. in rectus sheath	Muscular branches	To abdominal mm.
Pericardiophrenic a.	Internal thoracic a.	Accompanies phrenic n.	Pleura, pericardium, diaphragm	–	Pleura, pericardium, diaphragm

Table 2.4 Continued

Artery	Origin	Relations	Termination	Branches	Supply
Bronchial aa.	Two left bronchial aa. arise directly from the aorta. The single right bronchial a. arises from the third right posterior intercostal a.	Posterior thoracic wall	Small bronchial arteries supply the tissue of the lungs, bronchial tree and pulmonary pleura	–	Posterior thoracic wall, tissue of the lungs, bronchial tree and pulmonary pleura
Pulmonary trunk	R. ventricle	Divides under the arch of aorta into L. and R. pulmonary aa. Phrenic n. passes anterior and vagus posterior to trunks. Posterior + superior to pulmonary veins at the hilum **Right:** under arch of aorta to R. hilum. **Left:** anterior to descending aorta to L. hilum. At the bifurcation the L. pulmonary a. is joined by the ligamentum arteriosum entering the aorta (remnant of ductus arteriosum)	Hilum of the lung	Divides in the root of the lung to bronchopulmonary segments	Lungs

Table 2.4 Thoracic arteries (continued)

Artery	Origin	Relations	Termination	Branches	Supply
Ascending aorta	L. ventricle opposite third costal cartilage at left margin of sternum	Lies between the SVC and pulmonary trunk above the heart	Opposite second right costal cartilage at right margin of sternum	R. and L. coronary aa.	–
Arch of aorta	Opposite second R. costal cartilage	**Five things posterior and to the right:** trachea, oesophagus, L. recurrent n, thoracic duct, vertebral column **Five things anterior and to the left:** lung and pleura, L. phrenic, L. vagus, cardiac nerves, superior intercostal v. **Five things below:** L. bronchus, R. pulmonary artery, ligamentum arteriosum, L. recurrent laryngeal n., superficial cardiac plexus **Five things above:** L. common carotid a., L. subclavian v., brachiocephalic a., thymus, L. brachiocephalic v.	Left side of lower border of fourth thoracic vertebra	(Right) Brachiocephalic trunk L. common carotid L. subclavian	–

Table 2.4 Continued

Artery	Origin	Relations	Termination	Branches	Supply
Descending thoracic aorta	Left side of lower border of fourth thoracic vertebra	**Anterior:** root of left lung, oesophagus, left atrium, diaphragm **Posterior:** hemiazygos v., intercostal aa., longitudinal ligament of vertebra, L. lung and pleura **Right:** R. lung and pleura, oesophagus, azygos v., thoracic duct, dorsal vertebrae **Left:** hemiazygos v., L. lung, pleura, splanchnic nn.	Lower border of 12th dorsal vertebra, becoming abdominal aorta	Nine intercostals Four oesophageal Three bronchial Two diaphragmatic Mediastinal, pericardial and subcostal	–
Brachiocephalic trunk (arterial)	Opposite centre of manubrium from aortic arch	**Anterior:** thymus, L. brachiocephalic v., manubrium **Posterior:** trachea, lung and pleura **Right:** R. brachiocephalic v., SVC **Left:** L. common carotid a., trachea	Behind upper part of sternoclavicular joint by dividing into R. common carotid and R. subclavian	–	–

Table 2.4 Thoracic arteries (continued)

Artery	Origin	Relations	Termination	Branches	Supply
Subclavian a.	**Left:** from the aorta 1.25 cm below the sternoclavicular joint **Right:** from the bifurcation of the brachiocephalic trunk at the sternoclavicular joint	Course is divided into three parts by the scalenus anterior ***First part*** **Anterior:** Muscles – sternohyoid, sternothyroid Veins – internal jugular, anterior jugular Nerves – phrenic, vagus Structures – skin, superior fascia, platysma, deep fascia, common carotid, thoracic duct, right lymph duct **Posterior:** Lung, pleura, thoracic duct, longus cervicis. Oesophagus on the left. Recurrent laryngeal nerve on the right	On both sides at the lateral border of the first rib by becoming the axillary a.	(*Mnemonic:* VIT C+D) **V**ertebral **I**nternal thoracic **T**hyrocervical trunk: • Inferior thyroid • Transverse cervical • Suprascapular **C**ostocervical trunk: • Superior intercostal • Deep cervical	-

Table 2.4 Continued

Artery	Origin	Relations	Termination	Branches	Supply
		Third part **Below:** First rib **Above:** Transverse cervical artery Lowest trunk of brachial plexus **Posterior:** Lung and pleura Scalenus medius Lowest trunk of brachial plexus **Anterior:** Clavicle, platysma and subclavius, nerve to subclavius, external jugular v., anterior jugular, transverse cervical and suprascapular vv., skin, superficial, deep and pre-vertebral fascia, suprascapular a.			

Table 2.5 Thoracic veins

Vein	Origin	Relations	Termination	Tributaries
Internal thoracic w.	Superior epigastric v. + musculophrenic v.	Anterior to transversus thoracis just deep to the sternum	L. and R. brachiocephalic w.	
Intercostal w.	Intercostal muscles + skin	Accompany and lie above the arteries in neurovascular plane (between inner and innermost layers)	**Anterior:** drain to internal thoracic v. **Posterior:** drain to azygos + hemiazygos veins. First space ascend over neck of first rib and drain into the L. + R. brachiocephalic v.	
Pulmonary w.	Lung hila	Superior to coronary sinus Inferior to pulmonary arteries Anterior to descending aorta and pulmonary artery at hilum	Left atrium	
Bronchial w.	Lung parenchyma and pleura	Lie on posterior thoracic wall	Azygos or pulmonary w.	
Superior vena cava	Union of left and right brachiocephalic w.	Azygos v. joins near entry to R. atrium	Right atrium	

Table 2.5 Continued

Vein	Origin	Relations	Termination	Tributaries
Inferior vena cava	The intrathoracic course is very short Commences in front of the body of the fifth lumbar vertebra by union of the common iliac vv.	Central tendon of diaphragm to the right of midline at the level of T8 Fills R. cardiodiaphragmatic recess	Pierces the diaphragm opposite eighth thoracic vertebra and ends piercing pericardium in lower posterior part of right atrium	Phrenic – right Adrenal – right Renal – right Testicular – right Lumbars (third and fourth) Common iliacs Hepatics
Azygos v.	Abdominal contributions	Lies on the right posterior thoracic wall in the posterior mediastinum Contributions by intercostal vv. Contributions by the L. hemiazygos v. Enters thoracic cavity in relation to the R. crus Thoracic duct lies medially Sympathetic chain lies laterally	Enters SVC near its entry to R. atrium at T4	

Table 2.5 Thoracic veins (continued)

Vein	Origin	Relations	Termination	Tributaries
Hemiazygos v.	Abdominal contributions	Lies on the left posterior thoracic wall in the posterior mediastinum Contributions by intercostal veins Thoracic duct lies medially Sympathetic chain lies laterally	At azygos v.	
Brachiocephalic v.	Commences at the clavicle below the first costal cartilage by the union of the subclavian and internal jugular vv.	Left: longer course anterior to R. brachiocephalic a., L. common carotid a., and L. subclavian a., trachea Vagus and phrenic nerve are posterior Internal thoracic and inferior thyroid veins drain directly to brachiocephalic veins Lies in the superior mediastinum	Superior vena cava	
Subclavian v.	Lateral border of first rib as a continuation of the axillary v.	Anterior to scalenus anterior	Combines with internal jugular to form the brachiocephalic v.	Axillary vein and upper limb vv.

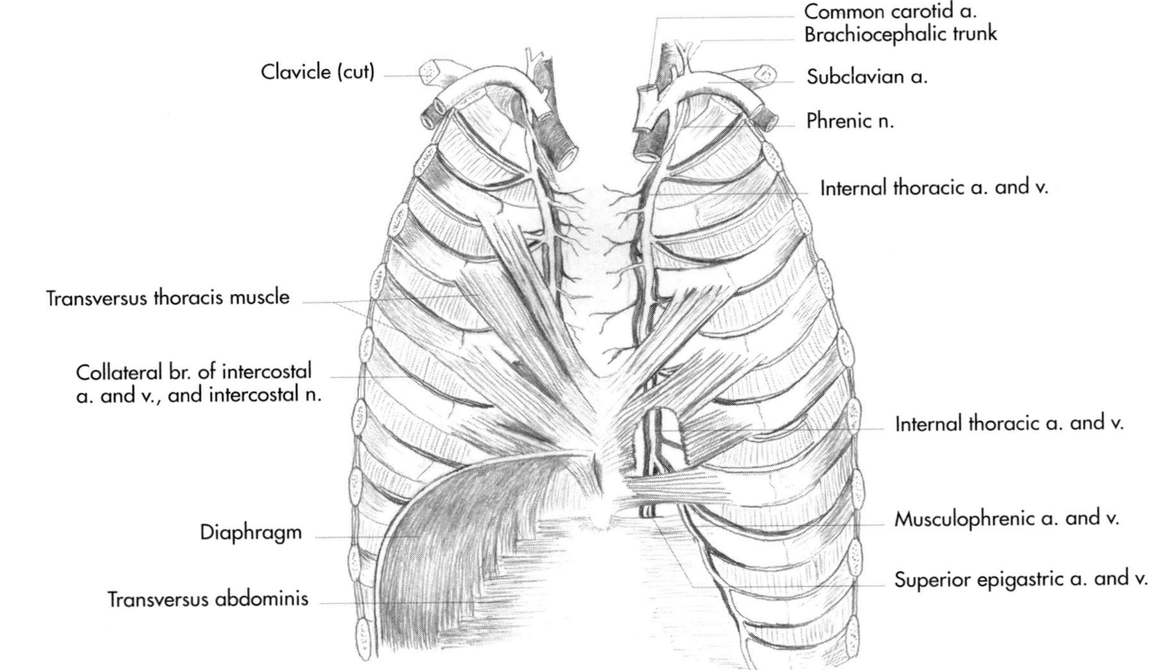

Figure 2.2 Internal view of anterior thoracic wall

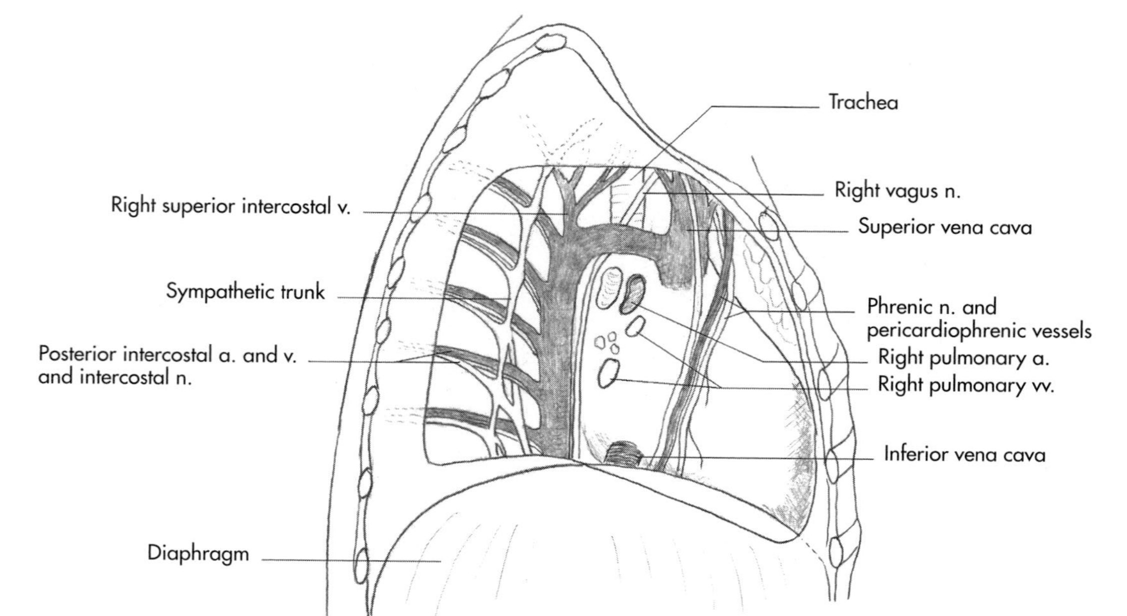

Figure 2.3 Right lateral view of mediastinum

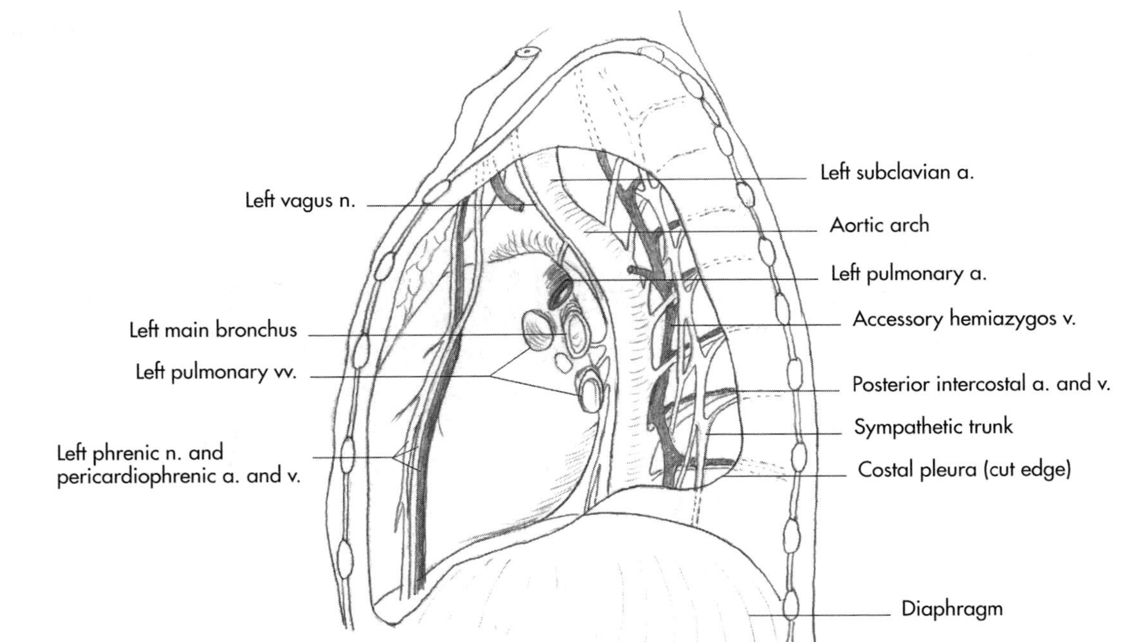

Figure 2.4 Left lateral view of mediastinum

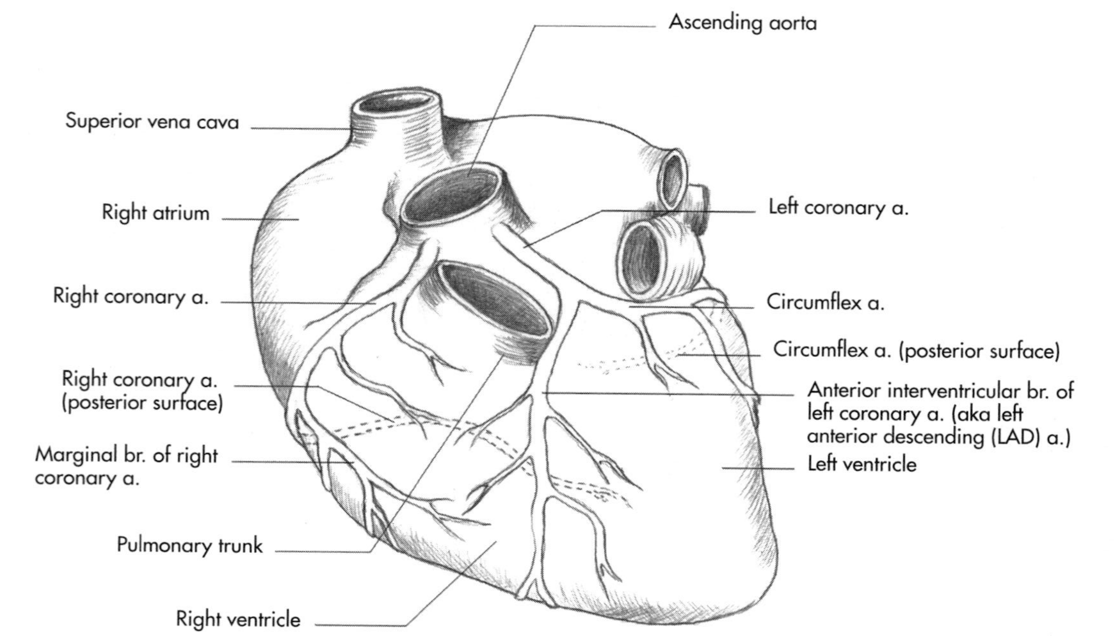

Figure 2.5 The heart and its blood supply

CHAPTER 3: ABDOMEN, PELVIS AND GENITOURINARY SYSTEM

ANTERIOR ABDOMINAL WALL

What is the innervation of the abdominal wall?	Ventral rami of T7–L1 (iliohypogastric nerve). These become superficial over the lateral aspect of the wall.
What is the abdominal reflex?	It is elicited by oblique strokes towards the umbilicus on the abdominal wall. Each stroke produces a brisk contraction of the underlying muscle. If this is absent think of an upper motor neurone lesion.
What is caput medusa?	This is the sign of dilated veins on the abdomen. It is caused by inferior vena cava obstruction (cirrhosis, thrombus, tumour). Communication develops between the portal veins and veins of the anterior abdominal wall (thoracoepigastic, intercostal and superficial epigastric veins).
What are the layers of the abdominal wall?	Skin. Superficial fascia (composed of adipose tissue). Deep membranous layer (Scarpa's fascia). Three layers of abdominal muscles or their fascia. Transversalis fascia. Parietal peritoneum.
What is the significance of the L1 plane?	Very important anatomical landmark! The following are found at this level: fundus of the gallbladder (at the point where this plane transects the ninth costal cartilage) pylorus of the stomach termination of the spinal cord

hila of kidneys and the renal vessels, which enter and leave
body of pancreas
splenic vein.
(*Synonym:* Addison's or transpyloric plane.)

How do you describe the transpyloric plane clinically?

As an imaginary horizontal line drawn through the midpoint of a line connecting the suprasternal notch to the symphysis pubis.

What are the nine subdivisions of the abdomen?

1. Left hypochondrium.
2. Epigastrium.
3. Right hypochondrium.
4. Left flank.
5. Periumbilical.
6. Right flank.
7. Left iliac fossa.
8. Suprapubis.
9. Right iliac fossa.

What lines divide it so?

Two vertical lines drawn from the midclavicular point to the midinguinal point.
Two horizontal lines:
the transpyloric plane
a line drawn through the tubercles of the iliac crests of the pelvis (transtubercular plane).
Intercristal plane: highest point of iliac crests (L4), important for lumbar punctures.

Where do hernias most commonly occur?

At areas of weakness in the abdominal wall (both anteriorly and posteriorly).
Anteriorly:
inguinal canal: inguinal hernias (direct at external [superficial] ring; indirect at internal [deep] ring)
femoral canal: femoral hernias
umbilical cicatrix (scar): umbilical (defect in cicatrix itself) or

paraumbilical (defect just lateral to cicatrix)
epigastric portion of linea alba: epigastric hernias
arcuate line of rectus sheath: spigelian hernias.

Posteriorly:
lumbar triangle (formed by free border of external oblique and iliac crest): lumbar hernias.

Also: obturator canal of the pelvis – obturator hernias.

What are the tendinous intersections?

One lies at the level of the umbilicus and two above. They are adherent to the anterior rectus sheath.

How is the rectus sheath formed?

It encloses rectus abdominis and is formed by the aponeurotic tendons of the external and internal oblique and transversus abdominis muscles. The external oblique aponeurosis passes anteriorly, and the internal aponeurosis splits in two with parts passing both anteriorly and posteriorly to the rectus muscle. The transversus aponeurosis passes posteriorly. Distal to the arcuate line (midway between the umbilicus and symphysis pubis) all aponeuroses pass anteriorly to the rectus abdominus muscle. Only the transversalis fascia lies posteriorly here.

INGUINAL REGION

Where does the inguinal ligament (of Poupart) run?

From the anterosuperior iliac spine (ASIS) to the pubic tubercle (approximately 1.5 cm lateral to the symphysis pubis).

What is the midinguinal point?

The midpoint of an imaginary line joining the ASIS to the symphysis pubis. This differs from the midpoint of the inguinal ligament, which is slightly lateral (one finger-breadth) to the midinguinal point.

What is the relevance of these two points?

2 cm below the midinguinal point is the anatomical landmark of:

the femoral artery

the femoral head.

The midpoint of the inguinal ligament is the anatomical landmark of the internal (or deep) ring of the inguinal canal.

What is the clinical significance of the pubic tubercle?

It is the anatomical landmark of the external (or superficial) ring.

What is the significance of the deep and superficial rings?

They are the entry and exit points, respectively, of the inguinal canal. The testis entered the canal via the deep ring and the scrotum via the superficial ring during its descent, dragging the spermatic cord behind it. This, in turn, was dragged by the gubernaculum, which attaches it to the scrotum.

What are the boundaries of the inguinal canal?

Anterior wall formed by the external oblique aponeurosis, assisted laterally by the internal oblique muscle.

Posterior wall is the conjoint tendon medially and the transversalis fascia throughout.

Roof is the lower edge of internal oblique and transversus muscles, which medially join together as the conjoint tendon and insert onto the pubic crest and the pectineal line of the pubic bone.

Floor is the in-rolled lower edge of the inguinal ligament, reinforced medially by the lacunar ligament.

What lies within the inguinal canal?

Males: spermatic cord.
Females: round ligament.

What are the contents of the spermatic cord?

Three arteries:
1. Testicular artery (from aorta).
2. Artery to ductus (vas) deferens (from superior vesical artery).
3. Cremasteric artery (from inferior epigastric artery).

Three nerves:
1. Genital branch of genitofemoral nerve.
2. Ilioinguinal nerve (lies on the cord).
3. Sympathetic nerves.

Four others:
1. Pampiniform plexus (testicular venous drainage).
2. Ductus (vas) deferens.
3. lymphatics.
4. Processus vaginalis (when bowel pushes into this it becomes the hernial sac).

What are the coverings of the spermatic cord?

Three in all, each derived during testicular descent.
From inside out:
1. Internal spermatic fascia: derived from the transversalis fascia at the deep inguinal ring.
2. Cremasteric fascia and muscle: derived from the internal oblique and transversus fascia and muscles.
3. External spermatic fascia: derived from the external oblique aponeurosis.

What is the drainage of the pampiniform plexus of veins?

The plexus condenses to three or four vessels that ascend through the inguinal canal to enter the inferior vena cava on the right and the left renal vein on the left, leading to the potential for varicocele formation.

Where do the lymphatics of the scrotum drain to?

They run alongside the testicular artery to the aortic nodes.

What is the difference between congenital and acquired inguinal hernias?

A **congenital** (indirect) hernia occurs when the process vaginalis fails to close in childhood, allowing the scrotum to be continuous with the peritoneal cavity via the spermatic cord. This predisposes the scrotum to become filled with peritoneal fluid or even bowel.

An **acquired** (direct) hernia occurs in later life as a result of a weakness in the abdominal wall, predisposed to by increased intra-abdominal pressure (e.g. in lifting). The weakness is at the posterior abdominal wall and the superficial ring. Contents do not enter the scrotum.

What is the certain way to make the correct hernia diagnosis?

If the clinical picture is unclear it can be differentiated by the location of the inferior epigastric artery. The deep ring through which the indirect hernia propagates lies lateral to the artery. A direct inguinal hernia will be medial to the artery. Doppler ultrasonography might be required to ascertain this.

What is the round ligament?

It is a remnant of the gubernaculum in the female. It extends from the ovary and passes along the inguinal canal to the labium majus.

What is Hesselbach's triangle?

A triangle on the inner surface of the abdominal wall through which direct inguinal hernias protrude. It is bounded laterally by the inferior epigastric artery, medially by the rectus muscle and inferiorly by the inguinal ligament. The conjoint tendon and the transversalis fascia stretch across the triangle.

How do obstruction, strangulation and incarceration of a hernia differ?

Obstruction: constriction of the lumen causing occlusion of the lumen.
Incarceration: obstruction causing an irreducible sac.
Strangulation: incarceration compromising venous return, causing venous **congestion**, arterial occlusion and gangrene. Peritonitis can ensue.

What are a herniorrhaphy and herniotomy?

Herniorrhaphy: a hernia repair with restoration of the normal anatomy of the weakened wall.
Herniotomy: a hernia repair performed on infants to repair an inguinal hernia. The patent processus vaginalis is ligated and excised.

FEMORAL CANAL

What are the boundaries of the femoral ring?

The femoral ring opens into the femoral canal:

- **laterally:** femoral vein
- **medially:** lacunar ligament (sharp, crescentic)
- **anteriorly:** inguinal ligament (of Poupart)
- **posteriorly:** pectineus muscle and its overlying fascia.

How can the arrangements of the contents of the femoral canal be remembered?

(*Mnemonic:* from lateral hip towards medial – NAVEL.)
Nerve (directly behind sheath).
Artery (within sheath).
Vein (within sheath).
Empty space (between vein and lymph).
Lymphatics (with deep inguinal node).
The nerve, artery and vein are all called 'femoral'.

PERITONEAL CAVITY

What is the epiploic foramen?

The opening from the greater sac of the peritoneal cavity into the lesser sac. (*Synonym:* foramen of Winslow.)

What is the lesser sac also known as?

The omental bursa.

What are the boundaries of the epiploic foramen?

Anteriorly: free border of the lesser omentum.
Posteriorly: Inferior vena cava.
Superiorly: caudate process of the liver.
Inferiorly: first part of the duodenum (D1).

What important structures lie within the free border of the omentum?

The following three:

- hepatic artery
- hepatic portal vein
- common bile duct.

How can bleeding secondary to a liver haemorrhage or a bloody open cholecystectomy be controlled at laparotomy?

By squeezing the free border of the omentum (and hence the hepatic artery) between your forefinger and thumb (Pringle's manoeuvre).

What are the walls of the lesser sac?

Anteriorly: liver, stomach, lesser omentum and greater omentum.
Posteriorly: diaphragm.
Right limit: oesophagus.
Left limit: spleen.

What lies in the lienorenal ligament?

The tail of the pancreas and the splenic vessels.

What are the differences between the median and the medial umbilical ligaments?

The **median ligament** is the fibrous remnant of the urachus, the fetal connection between the apex of the bladder and the umbilicus.
The **medial ligaments** are fibrous remnants of the fetal umbilical arteries, which arose from the internal iliacs.

What are the supracolic and infracolic compartments?

These are divided by the greater omentum. The supracolic cavity lies above the stomach. If the greater omentum is reflected back and upwards the infracolic compartment is exposed.

What are the folds on the deep aspect of the anterior abdominal wall (when viewed from within the abdominal cavity)?

Median umbilical fold: contains urachus.
Medial umbilical folds: contain obliterated umbilical arteries.
Lateral umbilical folds: contain inferior epigastric arteries.

What is the pelvic mesocolon?

An inverted V-shaped mesentery which attaches the sigmoid colon to the posterior abdominal wall.

What is it clinically useful as?

Its apex points to the divergence of the left common iliac artery.
The left ureter runs behind it.
The right limb runs to the midline of the third sacral vertebra.
The left limb descends along the medial border of the left psoas muscle.

STOMACH

Name the parts of the stomach.

See Figure 3.1.

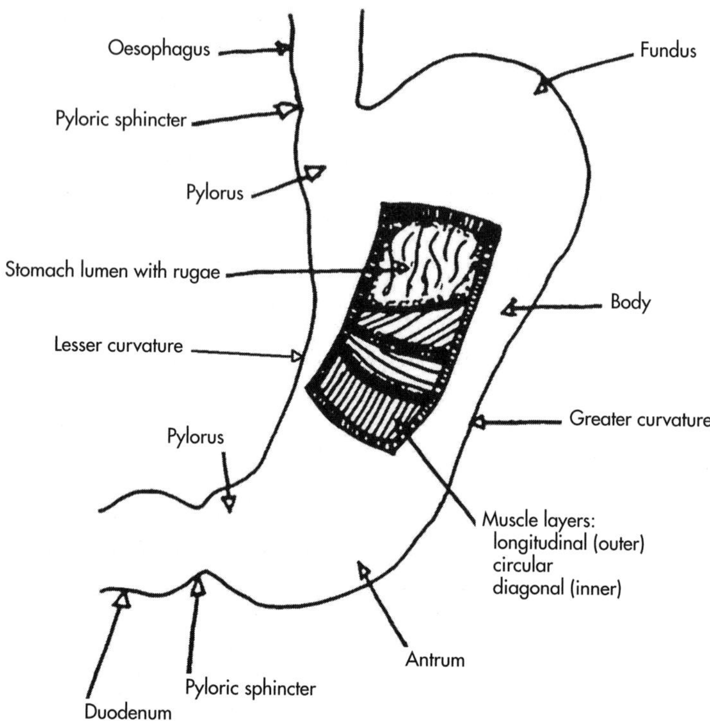

Figure 3.1

What is the origin of the stomach's blood supply?

The coeliac trunk, a branch of the abdominal aorta.

What comprises the stomach bed?

Upper part of left kidney.
Pancreas.
Spleen.
Left adrenal gland.
Transverse mesocolon.
Splenic artery.

Abdominal aorta.
Coeliac trunk and its branches.
Coeliac ganglion.
Coeliac lymph nodes.
Diaphragm (left crus and dome).
These structures are covered by the lesser sac, which lies between them and the posterior wall of the stomach.

SMALL BOWEL

What are the parts of the small bowel?

Duodenum, jejunum and ileum.

What part of the duodenum is retroperitoneal?

All but the first 1 cm lies retroperitoneally and is firmly attached to the posterior abdominal wall. The subsequent jejunum does not.

What is the blood supply of the duodenum?

Superior pancreaticoduodenal artery from the gastroduodenal artery of the hepatic artery.
Inferior pancreaticoduodenal artery from the superior mesenteric artery.

What are the lengths of each part of the duodenum?

(*Mnemonic:* count 1 to 4, but staggered)
D1 = 2 inches (5 cm).
D2 = 3 inches (7.5 cm).
D3 = 4 inches (10 cm).
D4 = 1 inch (2.5 cm).

How do you distinguish between jejunum and ileum at laparotomy?

See Table 3.1. (see overleaf)

What special functions does the intrinsic terminal ileum have?

1. Absorption of vitamin B_{12} (factor-dependent).
2. Absorption of bile salts (forms part of the enterohepatic circulation).

Table 3.1

	Jejunum	**Ileum**
Length (about 6 m [20 feet] in total)	About 2.5 m (8 feet]	About 4 m (12 feet)
Wall	Thick and double-walled (mucosa can be felt as a separate layer: 'shirt sleeve through a coat sleeve')	Thin and single-walled
Colour	Paler	Darker (as richer blood supply)
Vascular arcades (mesenteric arterial loops)	One to two arcades seen	Three to five arcades seen
Peyer's patches (lymphoid follicles on antimesenteric border)	Sparse	Numerous

COLON, RECTUM AND ANAL CANAL

Name the parts of the colon.

From proximal to distal: caecum → ascending colon → transverse colon → descending colon → sigmoid colon → rectum.

What are the distinguishing features of the caecum?

The small bowel empties into it via the ileocolic junction (usually guarded by the ileocaecal valve) and it bears the appendix.

What are the features that distinguish the colon from the small bowel?

1. Haustrae.
2. Taeniae coli.
3. Appendices epiploicae (fat appendages).

These are all found on the colon's external surface, whereas the small bowel is smooth and featureless.

How many parts is the rectum divided into?

Three, based on their blood supply and venous drainage.

What is the blood supply of the colon?

Mainly branches from the superior and inferior mesenteric arteries (SMA and IMA respectively):

- caecum: ileocolic artery (SMA)
- ascending colon: right colic artery (SMA)
- transverse colon: middle colic artery (SMA)
- descending colon: left colic artery (IMA)
- sigmoid colon: sigmoidal arteries (IMA).

And of the rectum?

Proximal third: superior rectal artery (branch of IMA).
Middle third: middle rectal artery (branch of internal iliac artery).
Distal third: inferior rectal artery (branch of pudendal artery, also a branch of the internal iliac artery).

What is the venous drainage of the colon?

The veins parallel the arteries and have similar names. They all ultimately drain into the portal vein.

And of the rectum?

Proximal third: inferior mesenteric vein → splenic vein → portal vein.
Middle and distal third: iliac vein (IVC).

What is the marginal artery of Drummond?

Artery formed by the anastomosis of the ileocolic, middle colic, right and left colic arteries, and the sigmoidal arteries. It is a continuous vessel running along the inner perimeter of the large intestine from the ileocolic junction to the rectum.

What is its clinical significance?

It is one of two tenuous blood supplies to the splenic flexure of the transverse colon, an area that is prone to bowel ischaemia because of this tenuous blood supply.

What is the other supply?

The anastomosis of the middle colic artery of the SMA and the upper left colic artery of the IMA.

What is the anal canal?

There are two definitions:

1. The surgical anal canal is approximately 4 cm long and extends from the anal verge or intersphincteric groove distally to the anorectal ring proximally
2. The anatomical anal canal is only approximately 2 cm long and extends from the anal verge distally to the dentate line proximally.

What is normally palpable on a rectal exam?

Both sexes: rectal mucosa, parasacral lymph nodes (if enlarged) and tip of coccyx.
Males: prostate and seminal vesicles anteriorly.
Female: upper third of vagina and cervix anteriorly.

How long is the anal canal?

4 cm.

What is its blood supply?

Upper end: superior rectal artery.
Lower end and mucosa: inferior rectal artery.
Also receives supply from the middle rectal and median sacral arteries.

What is its venous drainage?

Superior rectal vein, which drains the upper part and is continuous with the rectal venous plexus, and then on to the inferior mesenteric and portal veins.
Inferior and middle rectal veins, which drain the lower part into the internal iliac vein and then on to the IVC.
The anal canal is therefore a site of portosystemic anastomosis.

Where does this anastomosis occur?

At the anal cushions, spongy mucosal cushions that occur at 3, 7 and 11 o'clock (in the lithotomy position).

What else are these anal cushions important for?

They help maintain continence of flatus and keep the anal canal watertight.

Which sphincters control the anus?

Internal (under involuntary control) and external (under voluntary control).

What is the nerve supply of the anal canal?

Somatic: inferior rectal branches (S2) of the pudendal nerve supply the external sphincter and sensory supply of the lower end of the canal (hence painful conditions of the anus are registered via this nerve, and the external sphincter is under voluntary control).
Autonomic: supply the internal sphincter and upper end.
Sympathetic supply (pelvic plexus) causes contraction and parasympathetic supply (pelvic splanchnic nerve) causes relaxation (hence upper anal canal is insensate and under involuntary control).

What anatomical landmark divides the sensory parts of the anal canal?

The dentate line: above this line is insensate; below this line is cutaneous and registers pain.

What is the dentate line also a landmark for?

The anal valves: these contain submucosal glands, some of which penetrate into the internal sphincter. Infection of these glands can result in abscesses ± fistulae.

APPENDIX

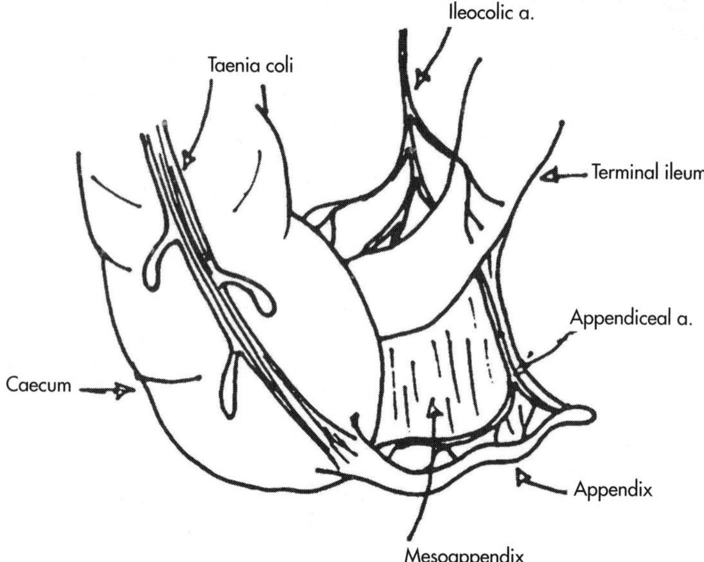

Figure 3.2

Where is the appendix? Attached to the end of the caecum.

What is its usual position? The posteromedial position.

What is its blood supply? The appendiceal artery, a branch of the ileocolic artery.

Where does it run? The free edge of the mesoappendix (mesentery of the appendix).

What is McBurney's point? The junction of the lateral and middle thirds of a line joining the anterosuperior iliac spine to the umbilicus. It is the point at which it is most tender in acute appendicitis as a result of irritation of the parietal peritoneum.

LIVER

What are the lobes of the liver?

It has four lobes: right, left, quadrate and caudate.
The large right lobe is separated from the smaller left lobe by a deep fissure. The quadrate and caudate lobes are seen posteriorly.

What is the liver's blood supply?

The hepatic artery (branch of the coeliac plexus) and the portal vein. The hepatic artery delivers oxygenated blood from the lungs, whereas the hepatic portal vein delivers blood from the gut and gut derivatives. The liver is drained by the hepatic veins to the IVC.

Tell me about the inferior liver markings.

There's a hepatic 'H' on the inferior surface of the liver. One vertical stick of the H is the dividing line for anatomical right/left lobe and the other vertical stick is the divider for vascular halves. The stick that divides the liver into vascular halves is the one with the vena cava impression (as the vena cava carries blood, it is fortunate that it is the divider for the vascular halves).

What attaches the liver to the diaphragm and anterior abdominal wall?

The falciform ligament.

What lies within the falciform ligament?

The ligamentum teres (left umbilical vein remnant), which runs in its free edge.

What is the bare area of the liver?

An area located on the superior surface of the liver, and so called because it is devoid of peritoneal covering. It is triangular in shape.
Apex: right triangular ligament.

Sides: widely separated leaves of the coronary ligament.
Base: left margin of the IVC.

What is unique about the liver?

It has two afferent blood supplies: hepatic artery and portal vein, both of which enter the liver via the porta hepatis.

What is the porta hepatis?

Central region of the liver (posterior surface), which contains the hepatic artery, portal vein, lymphatic vessels and extrahepatic bile ducts.

What structures does the portal vein drain?

Small and large intestines, stomach, spleen, pancreas and gallbladder.

What is a portosystemic shunt?

An anatomical area where the portal system (portal vein and tributaries) and the systemic system (IVC and tributaries) anastomose.

Where do you know these to occur?

Six sites in all:
1. Umbilical vein (normally obliterated in the adult, where it is known as the ligamentum teres or round ligament, which runs in the free edge of the falciform ligament; anastomoses with epigastric vein [systemic]).
2. Gastro-oesophageal junction.
3. Retroperitoneal veins.
4. Diaphragmatic veins.
5. Rectal plexus (superior [portal] veins to middle and inferior [systemic] veins).
6. Splenic veins (portal to the short gastric veins [systemic]).

What are the liver's functions?

They are as follows:
1. Formation of proteins such as albumin, prothrombin and fibrinogen.
2. Formation of bile and bilirubin metabolism.

3. Metabolism and storage of carbohydrates.
4. Metabolism of fats and phospholipids.
5. Metabolism of amino acids, with the formation of urea.
6. Storage of vitamins B_{12} and A, iron and copper.
7. Detoxification of drugs and hormones.
(By knowing the function of the liver well, you can predict the signs/symptoms and blood test changes that can occur in liver damage or failure!)

BILIARY TREE

What are the parts of the biliary tree?

See Figure 3.3.

What does the common bile duct drain into?

Second part of the duodenum (D2) via the ampulla of Vater (a raised mound on the inner surface of the midportion of D2).

What controls bile release into the duodenum at the ampulla?

The sphincter of Oddi.

What is the blood supply of the gallbladder?

The cystic artery, a branch of the right hepatic artery.

What is Calot's triangle?

An anatomical landmark for the cystic artery, and possibly the right hepatic artery on its way to the liver. Its boundaries are:
1. The common hepatic duct.
2. The cystic duct.
3. The inferior edge of the liver.

What else is in Calot's triangle?

A lymph node (Calot's node).

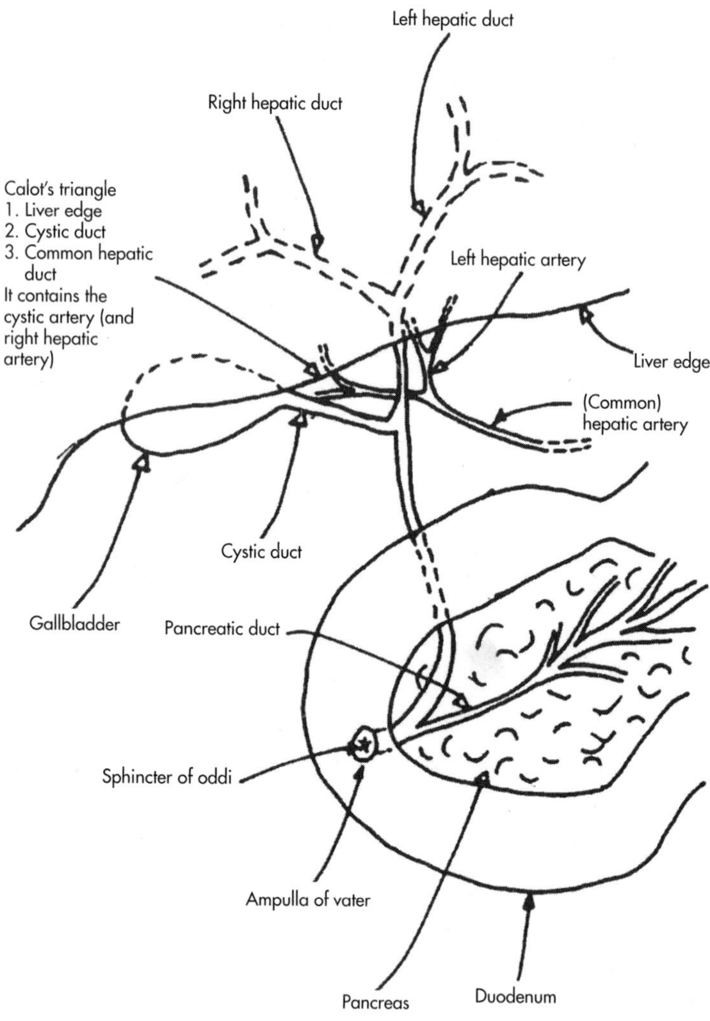

Figure 3.3

What is Hartmann's pouch? The infundibulum of the gallbladder (i.e. the portion of the gallbladder that meets the cystic duct).

What is its significance? It is the most common site of gallstone impaction.

Which liver enzyme is released by the biliary tree?

Alkaline phosphatase, which is therefore raised in biliary tree disease.

What does the gallbladder produce?

Mucus (not bile!).

PANCREAS

Where is the pancreas located?

In the retroperitoneum, forming part of the stomach bed.

What are its parts?

Head, uncinate process, neck, body and tail.

What is its blood supply?

Mainly from the splenic artery, but also contributions from the superior and inferior pancreaticoduodenal arteries (head); venous drainage via splenic vein (drains into portal vein).

What are its functions?

It is both an exocrine and an endocrine gland.
Exocrine: produces pancreatic juice containing trypsin, lipase and amylase (acinar glands), which aids in digestion.
Endocrine: produces glucagon (α cells) and insulin (β cells) from the islets of Langerhans located in the tail.

SPLEEN

How can the anatomy of the spleen be remembered?

By the odd numbers 3, 5, 7, 9, 11. Its dimensions are $3 \times 5 \times 7$ inches, and it lies posterior to the 9th to 11th left ribs.

What is its blood supply?

The splenic artery, one of the branches of the coeliac trunk of the abdominal aorta. Venous drainage is to the portal vein via the splenic and left gastroepiploic vv.

What type of organ is it?

A lymphoid organ with the following functions:

- filtration of red blood cells (RBCs)
- platelet storage
- opsonin production (important defence against encapsulated organisms, such as *Streptococcus pneumoniae*, meningococci, *Haemophilus influenzae* and *Escherichia coli*)
- phagocytosis (part of the reticuloendothelial system).

ABDOMINAL AORTA

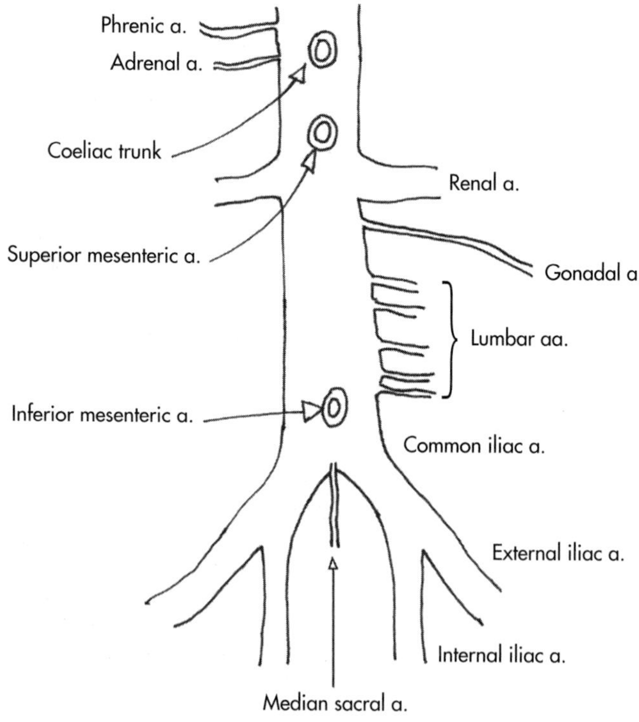

Figure 3.4

Which spinal levels does the aorta span?

T12 (behind median arcuate ligament) to L4.

What happens to it at L4?

Bifurcates into the left and right common iliac arteries.

Where is the aorta in relation to the IVC?

The aorta lies slightly to the left of the IVC.

Which renal artery is longer?

The right renal artery, as a result of the aorta being slightly displaced to the left.

What are the branches of the coeliac trunk?

1. Hepatic artery.
2. Left gastric artery.
3. Splenic artery.

What is the extent of the lower gastrointestinal tract?

From the ligament of Trietz to the anus.

What are the causes of lower gastrointestinal bleeding?

Altered blood:
1. Upper gastrointestinal bleed.
2. Right-sided colon neoplasm.

Fresh blood:
1. Haemorrhoids.
2. Diverticular disease.
3. Left-sided colon neoplasm.
4. Inflammatory bowel disease.
5. Angiodysplasia.
6. Ischaemic bowel.
7. Pseudomembranous colitis.
8. Infective causes, e.g. salmonellae.

PELVIS AND PERINEUM

What forms the hip bone?

Three bones:
1. Ilium.
2. Pubis.
3. Ischium.

At puberty the three bones are separated at the acetabulum by a Y-shaped piece of cartilage.

What are the differences between the male and female pelvis?

The acetabulum is larger in males. Its diameter is equal to the distance between its edge and the pubic symphysis. The male pelvis is deep and more conical. The female pelvis has a greater transverse diameter at the superior aperture.

What muscles form the floor of the pelvis?

It is a sling of a few muscles and referred to as the pelvic diaphragm.
Coccygeus (posteriorly).
Levator ani (anteriorly): pubococcygeus, iliococcygeus and puborectalis.

What does the pelvic floor support?

Males: urethra, prostate, bladder, rectum.
Females: urethra, bladder, vagina, rectum.

What is the lumbosacral trunk?

From L4 and L5 derivatives of the lumbar plexus, it connects the sacral plexus with the lumbar plexus. It descends at the medial border of the psoas muscle.

What is the urogenital diaphragm?

Found on the anterior aspect of the pelvic floor, it consists of a layer of striated muscle (deep transverse perineal muscles and sphincter urethra) sandwiched between two fascial layers (superior fascia of urogenital diaphragm and perineal membrane). The urethra passes through this diaphragm.

What else lies in the urogenital diaphragm?

Apart from the two muscles, the bulbourethral glands, the internal pudendal vessels and the dorsal nerves of the penis lie here.

Where does the perineal membrane lie?

It is a strong sheet of fascia spanning the two ischiopubic rami. Posteriorly it fuses and stops at the **perineal body** (central point for the

	attachment of the perineal musculature). It forms the inferior fascial layer of the urogenital diaphragm.
Why are these structures important?	When the urethra passes through the urogenital diaphragm it is called the membranous urethra. It is the perineal body that can be damaged during childbirth, causing incontinence of urine.
What are the ischioanal fossae?	Wedge-shaped, fat-filled spaces on either side of the anal canal. (*Synonym:* ischiorectal fossae, a misnomer.)
What are their boundaries?	Base: skin over anal region of perineum. Medial wall: anal canal and levator ani. Lateral wall: ischial tuberosity below and obturator internus muscle above. Apex: where the medial and lateral walls meet.
What is their significance?	Site of anorectal abscess formation.
Where is the pudendal canal and what lies in it?	It lies on the lateral wall of the ischiorectal fossa. It is deep to the perineal membrane just medial to the ischiopubic ramus. Within it are the pudenal nerve and internal pudendal vessels.

RENAL SYSTEM

What are the parts of the urinary tract?	See Figure 3.5.
What are the narrowest points?	Three points to remember: 1. Pelviureteric junction. 2. Point at which the ureter crosses the pelvic brim. 3. Vesicoureteric junction.

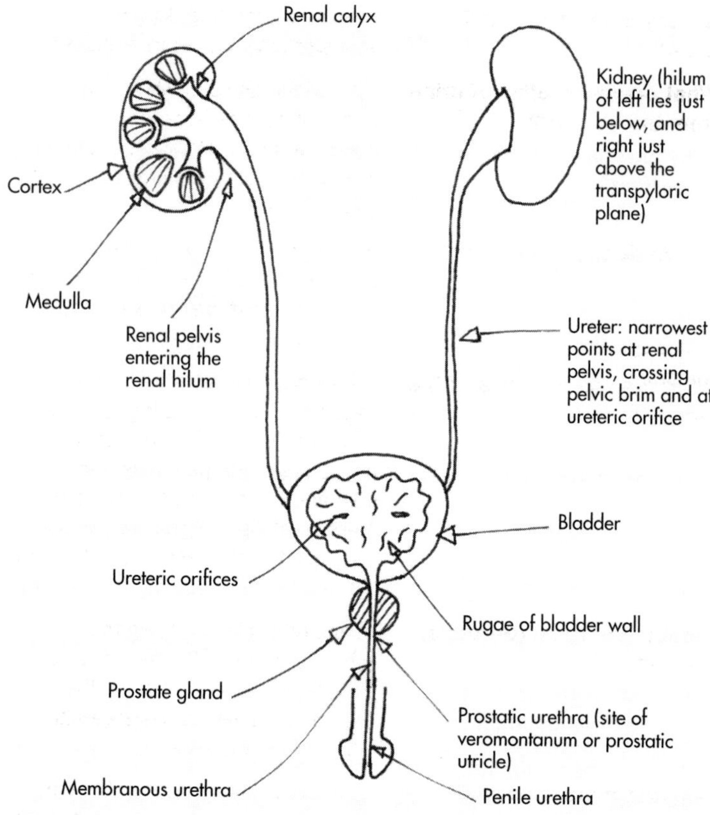

Figure 3.5

What is the clinical significance of this?	They represent the most common points that calculi can lodge and potentially cause urinary retention.
What is the diameter of the ureter?	Approximately 3 mm. Stones bigger than 3 mm in diameter will have a greater propensity to lodge (they can be measured on a radiograph). About 50% of calculi measuring 5 mm will pass.

So why is this important to know?

Stones greater than 3 mm in diameter may require intervention.

What prevents reflux of urine from the bladder?

The oblique angle at which the ureters enter the back into the ureters from the bladder at its trigone. This acts as a valve mechanism.

Where do the kidneys lie?

Roughly opposite L1–3 in the paravertebral gutters. They measure 12 cm in length and move with respiration.

What are the relations of the kidney?

The kidneys are retroperitoneal structures. Both the upper poles are related to the adrenal glands. The hila relate to the pancreas and duodenum. The colic flexures are anterior, along with the liver on the right and the stomach and spleen on the left.

What is the renal (Gerota's) fascia?

Layers of fascia enclosing the kidneys, perirenal fat and adrenal glands. They enclose part of the ureters and eventually merge with adjacent peritoneum.

Where are the glomeruli found?

The kidney receives about 20% of the cardiac output. The renal arteries divide into anterior and posterior branches, then segmental and interlobar arteries. These supply the glomeruli in the renal cortex.

What is the course of the ureters?

The ureters leave the hilum posterior to the blood vessels. They descend in the retroperitoneum on the surface of the psoas muscle over the sacroiliac joints. They cross over the iliac artery and, at the level of the ischial spines, turn medially into the base of the bladder.

What is the blood supply of the adrenal glands?

Branches of the inferior phrenic and renal arteries via the adrenal arteries. The outer cortex produces the corticosteroids and the inner medulla produces epinephrine (adrenaline) and norepinephrine (noradrenaline).

What is the bladder?

A distensible muscular organ lined with transitional epithelium lying on the pelvic floor and pubic symphysis. It stores urine.

When can the bladder be palpated?

The bladder needs to contain more than 300 ml before it can be palpated above the pubic symphysis. In chronic urinary retention it can have a capacity of over 1 litre and be palpable up to the umbilicus.

What is the trigone?

A triangular, smooth, reddish zone at the base. It is formed by two ureteric orifices and the internal urethral orifice.

What is the blood supply?

Superior and inferior vesical branches of the internal iliac arteries.

How does micturition occur?

Parasympathetic nerves are motor to the detrusor muscle but inhibit the internal sphincter. Sympathetic nerves inhibit the detrusor muscle. The external urethral sphincter is under voluntary control (pudendal nerve).

MALE REPRODUCTIVE SYSTEM

What are the stages of testicular descent?

Month 2: intra-abdominal structure.
End of month 4: testis at deep inguinal ring.
Month 7: within inguinal canal.
Shortly after birth: within scrotum.

What precedes the testis during descent?

The gubernaculum.

What is the gubernaculum?

A mesenchymal condensation attached to the inferior pole of the testis, the gradual contraction of which is thought to drag the testis behind it into the scrotum, where it eventually attaches.

In what does the testis descend?

A peritoneal invagination, the **processus vaginalis**.

What is the fate of the processus vaginalis?

Its lumen obliterates shortly after birth, leaving only a small portion surrounding the testis, the **tunica vaginalis**, attached to its posterior and lateral surfaces.

What is the clinical significance of the testes originating in the abdomen?

Two main reasons:
1. Testicular trauma (eg a kick) is felt in the abdomen (mainly periumbilical) caused by **referred pain**, the nerve supply of the testes being from T10.
2. Testicular cancer metastasises to the **para-aortic nodes**, and *not* the inguinal nodes like the scrotum (**an important concept and favourite exam question!**).

What is the penis made up of?

Two **corpora cavernosa** (singular corpus cavernosum), the erectile portions of the penis that abut the **glans penis**. The glans penis is the dilated end-part of the **corpus spongiosum**, which contains the penile urethra.

What type of epithelium is the penile urethra made up of?

Transitional cell epithelium for most of its length, except for its distal portion, which is squamous.

How can the layers of the scrotum be remembered?

(*Mnemonic:* **S**ome **D**amned **E**nglishman **C**alled **I**t **T**he **Testis**.)
Skin.
Dartos.
External spermatic fascia.

Cremasteric muscle.
Internal spermatic fascia.
Tunica vaginalis.
Testis.

What is the prostate gland?

A male organ attached to the bladder neck which forms the main bulk of ejaculate.

Can you describe it?

It is a chestnut-shaped gland approximately 20 g in weight in the normal adult male.

What is its structure?

It is composed of **epithelial** and **stromal** elements. Epithelial cells form acinar glands, whereas stroma forms collagen and smooth-muscle fibres.

What are different zones of the prostate?

Peripheral (70%), central (25%), transitional (5%).
Benign prostatic hypertrophy mainly develops in the **transitional zone**.

What is benign prostatic hypertrophy?

Benign prostatic hypertrophy mainly develops in the transitional zone and consists of hyperplasia of glandular and supporting tissue, mainly of the middle lobe. This causes obstruction at the bladder neck, consequently causing hypertrophy of the bladder because it must contract with greater force. The symptoms are known as lower urinary tract symptoms.

What is the anatomy of the ductus (vas) deferens?

From the epididymis through the spermatic cord and at the deep ring it hooks around the inferior epigastric vessels and crosses over the external iliac vessels to enter the pelvis. It crosses over the ureter ('bridge over water') to enter the prostate and urethra.

FEMALE REPRODUCTIVE SYSTEM

What are the contents of the broad ligament?

The broad ligament is a double layer of peritoneum hanging down over the uterus and associated structures:

- fallopian tube
- ovarian artery (branch of aorta)
- suspensory ligament of the ovary
- ligament of the ovary
- ovary
- round ligament
- uterine artery (branch of internal iliac)
- cardinal ligament (transverse cervical).

How can the contents of the broad ligament be remembered?

(*Mnemonic:* **BROAD**.)
Bundle (ovarian neurovascular bundle).
Round ligament.
Ovarian ligament.
Artefacts (vestigial structures).
Duct (oviduct).

What is the uterus?

A thick-walled, muscular cavity lined with endometrium (mucous membrane). It is continuous with the vagina via the cervix. It measures $3 \times 2 \times 1$ inches in the virgin state. It is divided into three parts:

1. Fundus.
2. Body.
3. Cervix.

What is the pouch of Douglas?

The rectouterine pouch.

What parts of the vagina are related to peritoneum?

Posterior vaginal fornix. This is a possible site for intra-abdominal abscess drainage.

Table 3.2 Anterior abdominal wall muscles

Muscle	Origin	Insertion	Action	Innervation
External oblique	Lower eight ribs' outer surface Free posterior margin	Linea alba Outer margin of iliac crest Inguinal ligament	Run downwards and medially	Intercostal nn. Lumbar spinal nn.
Internal oblique	Thoracolumbar fascia Deep to external oblique	Costal margin Linea alba	Run backwards Elevate thoracic cavity in AP axis Increase transverse thoracic diameter	Intercostal n. Lumbar spinal nn.
Transversus abdominis	Deep surface of costal margin Thoracolumbar fascia Anterior two-thirds of iliac crest Lateral two-thirds of inguinal ligament	Linea alba	Run forwards Elevate thoracic cavity in AP axis Increase transverse thoracic diameter	Intercostal n. Lumbar spinal nn.
Rectus abdominis	Fifth, sixth and seventh costal cartilages medially	Pubic crest and symphysis	Trunk flexion	Intercostal n. Lumbar spinal n.
Pyramidalis	Anterior pubic ligament	Linea alba	Trunk flexion	Intercostal n. Lumbar spinal n

AP, anteroposterior.

Table 3.3 Posterior abdominal wall muscles

Muscle	Origin	Insertion	Action	Innervation
Psoas major	T12–L5 lumbar vertebrae Intervertebral discs	Lesser trochanter	Hip flexion	L1–3
Psoas minor	T12–L5 lumbar vertebrae Intervertebral discs	Lesser trochanter	Hip flexion	L1–2
Iliacus	Ala of iliac bone	Lesser trochanter	Hip flexion	Femoral n. L2–4
Quadratus lumborum	Lower border of 12th rib	Iliolumbar ligament – spanning from fifth lumber vertebra and iliac crest	Stabilises twelfth rib in inspiration Lateral flexor of trunk	T12–L3 segmental nn.

Table 3.4 Pelvic floor muscles

Muscle	Origin	Insertion	Action	Innervation
Coccygeus	Ischial spine	Lateral margin of lower sacrum and coccyx	Pelvic floor	S4
Levator ani	Inner aspect of body of pubis and obturator fascia (arcus tendinus)	Ischial spine	Pelvic floor	S4 pudendal n.
External anal sphincter	Anococcygeal ligament Puborectalis portion of levator ani	Perineal body	Voluntary sphincter control	S4 perineal branch of pudenal n.
Sphincter urethrae	Encircle the urethra	Perineal body	Voluntary sphincter control	S4 perineal branch of pudendal n.
Deep transverse perineal	Fascia of lateral wall of perineum	Tendinous raphe and perineal body	Sphincter control	S4 perineal branch of pudendal n.

Table 3.5 Abdominal and pelvic nerves

Nerve	Source	Course and relations	Branches	Type
Lumbar plexus	Spinal cord	Lies in the substance of the psoas muscle. The nerves emerge from the margins	Related to psoas **Lateral aspect:** • Iliohypogastric • Ilioinguinal • Lateral femoral cutaneous nerve of the thigh • Femoral **Anterior surface:** • Genitofemoral **Medial aspect:** • Obturator	(See branches below)
Pelvic splanchnic nn. (parasympathetic)	S1–4 ventral rami Pelvic parasympathetic outflow	To various plexuses	Abdominal and pelvic plexus	Motor: pelvic viscera, large bowel beyond distal third of transverse colon
Iliohypogastric n.	L1	Lateral border of psoas, over posterior abdominal wall, then penetrates transversus abdominis to enter the neurovascular plane. The kidney is found anterior to the nerve	Lateral and anterior iliohypogastrics	Motor: transversus abdominis, internal oblique Sensory: upper lateral thigh, lower abdomen above pubis

Table 3.5 Abdominal and pelvic nerves (continued)

Nerve	Source	Course and relations	Branches	Type
Ilioinguinal n.	L1	Around posterior abdominal wall and enters the neurovascular plane. Just above the deep inguinal ring it perforates and lies superficial to the external oblique and enters the inguinal canal below the spermatic cord. The kidney is found anterior to the nerve	–	Motor: transversus abdominis, internal oblique Sensory: scrotum – male, mons pubis – female; also inner thigh
Lateral femoral cutaneous n.	L2–3	Emerges from the lateral border of the psoas m. It runs over the iliacus m. to enter the thigh beneath the lateral end of the inguinal ligament	–	Sensory: lateral aspect of thigh
Genitofemoral n.	L1–2	Appears after protruding through the psoas muscle to lie on its surface. Here it descends, dividing into the genital and femoral branches. The genital branch joins the spermatic cord or round ligament in the female. The femoral n. branch passes deep to the femoral ligament on the lateral side of the external iliac and femoral arteries	Genital and femoral branches	**Genital:** Motor: cremaster Sensory: external genitalia, skin below inguinal ligament **Femoral:** Sensory: upper femoral triangle
Obturator n.	(See lower limb)			
Pudendal n.	L2–4	Passes out of the greater sciatic foramen and re-enters the pelvis back through the lesser sciatic foramen. Accompanies the internal pudendal artery across the lateral wall of the ischiorectal fossa in the pudendal canal	Inferior rectal Perineal Dorsal nerve of penis	Motor: striated muscles of perineum Sensory: scrotal and penile sensation

Table 3.6 Abdominal and pelvic arteries

Artery	Origin	Relations	Termination	Branches	Supply
Abdominal aorta	Lower margin of 12th thoracic vertebra	**Anterior:** Coeliac and aortic plexus Body and uncinate process of pancreas Splenic vein Third part of duodenum Peritoneum Small intestine **Posterior:** Lumbar vertebrae Longitudinal ligament Third and fourth L. lumbar veins **Right:** Right crus of diaphragm Inferior vena cava Azygos v. Cisterna chyli **Left:** Left ureter Left crus of diaphragm Sympathetic trunk Small intestine Peritoneum Terminal part of duodenum	Lower margin of fourth lumbar vertebra	**Unpaired:** Coeliac trunk Superior mesenteric a. Inferior mesenteric a. Median sacral a. (at bifurcation) **Paired (visceral):** Adrenal Renal Gonadal (ovarian/testicular) **Paired (abdominal wall):** Subcostal Inferior phrenic Lumbar (four on each side)	Various organs via branches (see below)

Table 3.6 Abdominal and pelvic arteries (continued)

Artery	Origin	Relations	Termination	Branches	Supply
Inferior phrenic aa.	Abdominal aorta soon after it enters the abdominal cavity	The left phrenic a. passes behind the oesophagus passing on to the diaphragm. The right passes behind the IVC and liver	Forms anastomosis with the musculophrenic (internal thoracic) and intercostal aa.	Suprarenal a.	Diaphragm (and adrenal glands)
Lumbar aa.	Four pairs from aorta	Pass behind the psoas m. and sympathetic trunk (and vena cava on the right)	Abdominal wall	Dorsal br. Abdominal br.	Posterior abdominal wall and lumbar vertebrae
Coeliac trunk	From the anterior abdominal aorta opposite the 12th thoracic vertebra	Below the caudate lobe of the liver at the upper border of the pancreas with a crus and a coeliac ganglion on each side. It lies behind the cavity of the lesser sac	Behind the lesser sac of the peritoneum by subdivision into its three branches	Left gastric a. Splenic a. Common hepatic a.	Various structures via its branches
Splenic a.	As a branch of the coeliac trunk	Along the posterior abdominal wall at the upper border of the spleen reaching the lienorenal ligament **Anterior:** Lesser sac Stomach Pancreas **Posterior:** Left crus Left coeliac ganglion Left adrenal gland Left kidney	At the hilum of the spleen by subdivision into five to eight branches	Pancreatic a. Left gastroepiploic a. Short gastric a.	Spleen, body and tail of pancreas, stomach

Table 3.6 Continued

Artery	Origin	Relations	Termination	Branches	Supply
Left gastric a.	As a branch of the coeliac trunk at T12	It ascends on the posterior abdominal wall to reach the gastro-oesophageal junction. It then descends to anastomose with the right gastric a.	Anastomosis with the right gastric artery on the lesser curvature of the stomach	Oesophageal Short gastric	Stomach, lower end of oesophagus
Common hepatic a.	As a branch of the coeliac trunk at T12	It crosses the posterior abdominal wall to the right until the retroperitoneal first part of the duodenum. Branches are given off, continuing as the proper hepatic artery. It is then carried to the liver in the free border of the lesser omentum. It the lies to the left of the common hepatic duct and anterior to the portal vein. As it approaches the porta hepatis it divides	At the porta hepatis by the subdivision into right and left hepatic branches	Right gastric a. Gastroduodenal a. ⇒ pancreaticoduodenal + right gastroepiploic aa. Right hepatic a. Left hepatic a. Cystic a. (usually from right)	Stomach, first part of duodenum, liver via its branches
Right gastric a.	From the common hepatic a.	Lesser curvature of the stomach	Anastomosis with the left gastric a.	Short gastric a.	Stomach
Gastroduodenal a.	From the common hepatic a. at the first part of the duodenum	It passes behind the duodenum	Divides into its terminal branches	Right gastroepiploic a. Superior pancreaticoduodenal a.	Stomach and first part of duodenum
Gastroepiploic aa.	Left and right aa. arise from the splenic and gastroduodenal aa. respectively	Greater curvature of the stomach	Anastomose with each other	Short gastric and omental branches	Stomach

Table 3.6 Abdominal and pelvic arteries (continued)

Artery	Origin	Relations	Termination	Branches	Supply
Superior pancreaticoduodenal aa.	Arise from the gastroduodenal a. as a single a. or as anterior and posterior vessels	The anterior and posterior arteries descend in front and behind the head of the pancreas	Anastomose with the inferior pancreaticoduodenal aa.	Duodenal and pancreatic branches	Duodenum and head of pancreas
Cystic a.	Usually a branch of the right branch of the hepatic a.	Passes behind the common bile duct in Calot's triangle	At the gallbladder	–	Gallbladder
Superior mesenteric a.	From the abdominal aorta in the transpyloric plane (L1), behind the pancreas	**Anterior:** Pancreas Splenic v. Mesentery Small intestine **Posterior:** Left renal v. Uncinate process of the pancreas Third part of duodenum IVC Testicular vessels Genitofemoral n. Psoas	In the right iliac fossa by continuing as the ileocolic a.	Inferior pancreatoduodenal a. Jejunal a. Middle colic a. Right colic a. Ileocolic a. ⇒ appendiceal a.	–

Table 3.6 Continued

Artery	Origin	Relations	Termination	Branches	Supply
Renal aa.	Opposite the second lumbar vertebra from the aorta	**Anterior:** *Right:* Second part of duodenum Renal v. Inferior vena cava Head of pancreas *Left:* Renal v. Inferior mesenteric v. Pancreas **Posterior:** Crus Psoas	Hilum of kidneys with a subdivision into three stems: two behind and one in front of the renal pelvis	Ureteric Inferior adrenal	Kidneys
Gonadal a.	Abdominal aorta just below the renal arteries at second lumber vertebra	Descends on the psoas mm. passing anterior to the ureters and the external iliacs to enter the pelvis, heading either to the ovaries or within spermatic cord to the posterior aspect of the testis	Testis/ovary	Cremasteric Ureteric Testicular Epididymal Perforates tunica albuginea to reach the testis	Testis/ovary
Inferior mesenteric a.	From the anterior aspect of the aorta at the third lumbar vertebra 4 cm above the bifurcation	**Posterior:** Fourth left lumbar vessels Left common iliac artery Sympathetic trunk Left psoas	Becomes the superior rectal artery in front of the common iliac artery	Upper left colic Lower left colic Superior rectal	–

Table 3.6 Abdominal and pelvic arteries (continued)

Artery	Origin	Relations	Termination	Branches	Supply
Common iliac aa.	At the lower border of the left side of the fourth lumbar vertebra from the bifurcation of the aorta	**Anterior:** Peritoneum Bowel Ureter Left colic vessels Superior rectal vessels **Posterior:** Psoas Sympathetic trunk Obturator n. Lumbosacral trunk	At the lumbosacral articulation by subdivision into external and internal iliacs	Internal and external iliac aa.	–
External iliac aa.	Commence at the lumbosacral articulation from the bifurcation of the common iliacs	Pass around the brim of the pelvis at the medial border of the psoas m. **Anterior:** Peritoneum Bowel Testicular vessels Ureter Genitofemoral n. Vas deferens Deep circumflex iliac v. **Posterior:** Psoas Obturator n. External iliac a.	At the distal boarder of the inguinal ligament, continuing as the femoral a.	Becomes femoral a. as it passes beneath the inguinal ligament	–

Table 3.6 Continued

Artery	Origin	Relations	Termination	Branches	Supply
Internal iliac aa.	Commence at the lumbosacral articulation from the bifurcation of the common iliacs	Enter the pelvic cavity posteriorly in front of the sacroiliac joints	At the upper margin of the great sciatic notch by subdivision into anterior and posterior divisions	**Anterior division:** Superior vesical a. Inferior vesical a. Middle rectal a. Obturator a. Internal pudendal a. Inferior gluteal a. Uterine a. Vaginal a. **Posterior division:** Superior gluteal a. Iliolumbar a. Lateral sacral a.	–
Internal pudendal a.	As a continuation of the anterior division of the internal iliac a., passes out of the greater back through the lesser sciatic foramen	Crosses the pelvic surface of the sacral plexus. It leaves through the greater sciatic foramen below the piriformis m. above the sacrospinal ligament. It then curves behind the ischial spine to enter the perineum via the lesser sciatic foramen	Terminal branches	Inferior rectal Posterior scrotal Artery of bulb Arteries of penis – dorsal and deep perineal	–

Table 3.6 Abdominal and pelvic arteries (continued)

Artery	Origin	Relations	Termination	Branches	Supply
Obturator a.	Anterior trunk of internal iliac a.	Around the lateral wall of the pelvis under the perineum onto the medial surface of the obturator internus m. it pierces the obturator muscle through the obturator canal with the obturator n. It is crossed medially by the ureter and ductus deferens	Anastomosis with pelvic aa. and arteries of the gluteal region	Iliac a. Vesical a. Divides into internal and external branches external to the obturator canal	–
Uterine a.	Internal iliac a.	Leaves the internal iliac on the wall of the pelvis, passing over the ureter into the base of the broad ligament at the level of the cervix. It then ascends towards the ovarian a.	Anastomosis with the ovarian and vaginal aa.	–	Uterus
Vaginal a. (inferior vesical a. in male)	Anterior trunk of internal iliac a.	It descends onto the vagina	Anastomosis with vaginal and uterine aa.	To the neck of the bladder	Vagina and neck of bladder
Vesical a.	Anterior trunk of internal iliac a.	The bladder wall	Anastomosis with other vesical aa. on the surface of the bladder	–	Bladder
Middle rectal a.	Anterior trunk of internal iliac a.	The rectum	Anastomosis with superior and inferior rectal aa.	–	Rectum

Table 3.6 Continued

Artery	Origin	Relations	Termination	Branches	Supply
Superior gluteal a.	Internal iliac a., posterior aspect	Exits greater sciatic foramen above the piriformis	Gluteal region	The superior gluteal a. is a continuation of the posterior trunk. It divides into superficial and deep branches and supplies the medius and minimus gluteal mm.	Gluteal maximus, piriform and tensor fascia lata
Iliolumbar a.	Internal iliac a., posterior aspect	Ascends beneath the psoas m.	Iliacus and psoas m.	Muscular br.	Iliacus and psoas mm.
Inferior gluteal (sciatic) a.	Terminal branch of the anterior trunk of the internal iliac a.	Passes inferiorly on the sacral plexus and the piriformis behind the internal pudendal a. to the lower part of the greater sciatic foramen, exiting between piriformis and coccygeus mm. It continues between the greater trochanter of the femur and tuberosity of the ischium accompanying the sciatic and posterior femoral cutaneous nn.	To muscles and skin in back of thigh	Muscular br. to gluteus maximus and back of thigh Coccygeal br.	Muscles and skin in back of thigh

Table 3.7 Abdominal and pelvic veins

Vein	Origin	Relations	Termination	Tributaries
Pampiniform plexus/testicular v.	Scrotum	Spermatic cord Plexus condenses to three or four veins and ascends through the inguinal canal. Condenses to one vein as the testicular vein	**Right:** IVC **Left:** L. renal vein	
Superficial epigastric v.	Anterior abdominal wall	Anterior to rectus sheath	Inferior epigastric	
Portal v.	Behind the neck of pancreas by the union of splenic and superior mesenteric veins opposite the first lumbar vertebra	Runs from behind the neck of the pancreas and behind the pylorus into the free edge of the lesser omentum along with the common bile duct and hepatic artery	At the porta hepatis of the liver, subdividing into the right and left branches, each of which break up into capillaries around the liver lobules	Contributions from: Spleen Gallbladder Pancreas Peritoneum Large and small bowel Stomach

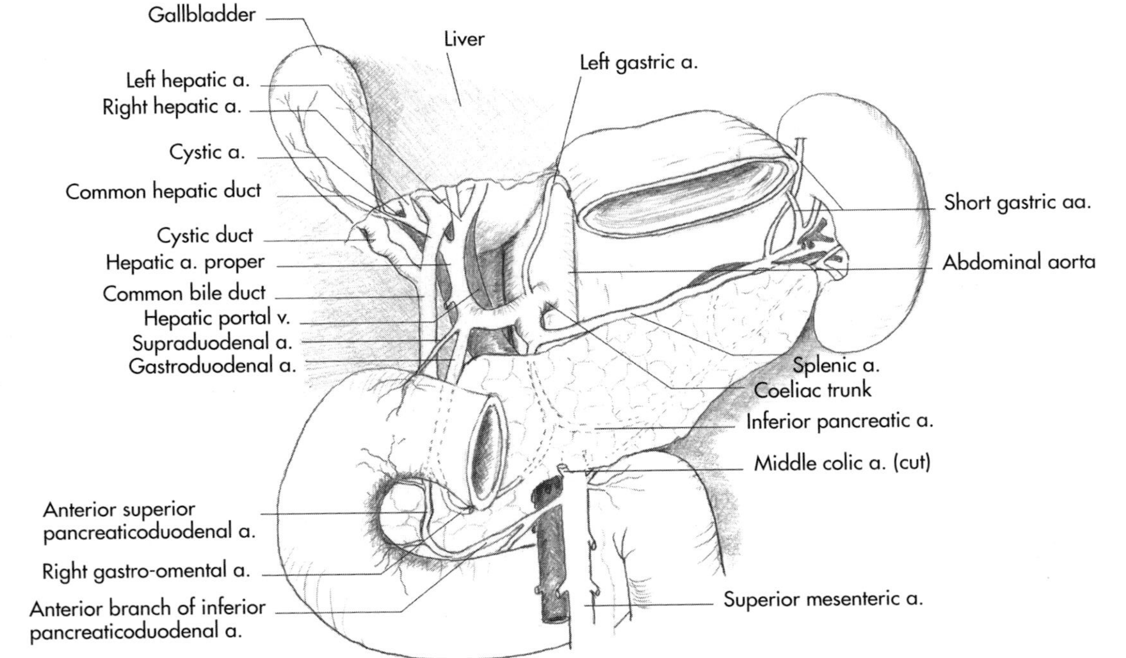
Gallbladder
Liver
Left gastric a.
Left hepatic a.
Right hepatic a.
Cystic a.
Common hepatic duct
Short gastric aa.
Cystic duct
Hepatic a. proper
Abdominal aorta
Common bile duct
Hepatic portal v.
Supraduodenal a.
Gastroduodenal a.
Splenic a.
Coeliac trunk
Inferior pancreatic a.
Middle colic a. (cut)
Anterior superior
pancreaticoduodenal a.
Right gastro-omental a.
Anterior branch of inferior
pancreaticoduodenal a.
Superior mesenteric a.

Figure 3.6 Upper gastrointestinal tract

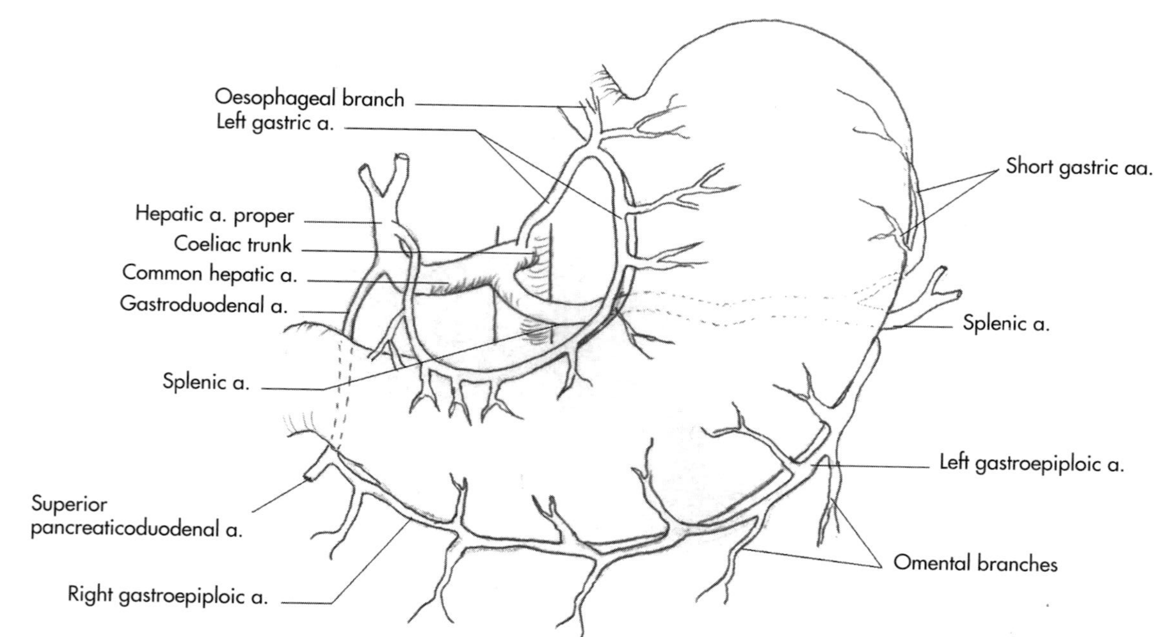

Figure 3.7 Gastric blood supply

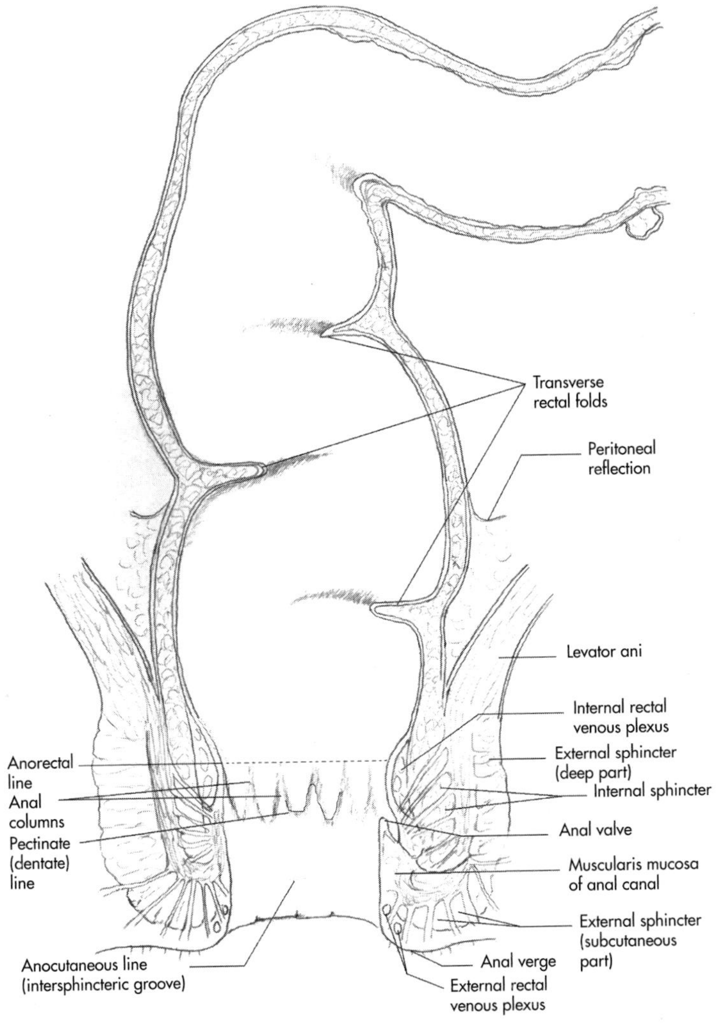
Transverse
rectal folds
Peritoneal
reflection
Levator ani
Internal rectal
venous plexus
External sphincter
(deep part)
Internal sphincter
Anal valve
Muscularis mucosa
of anal canal
External sphincter
(subcutaneous
part)
Anal verge
External rectal
venous plexus
Anorectal
line
Anal
columns
Pectinate
(dentate)
line
Anocutaneous line
(intersphincteric groove)

Figure 3.8 Rectum and anal canal

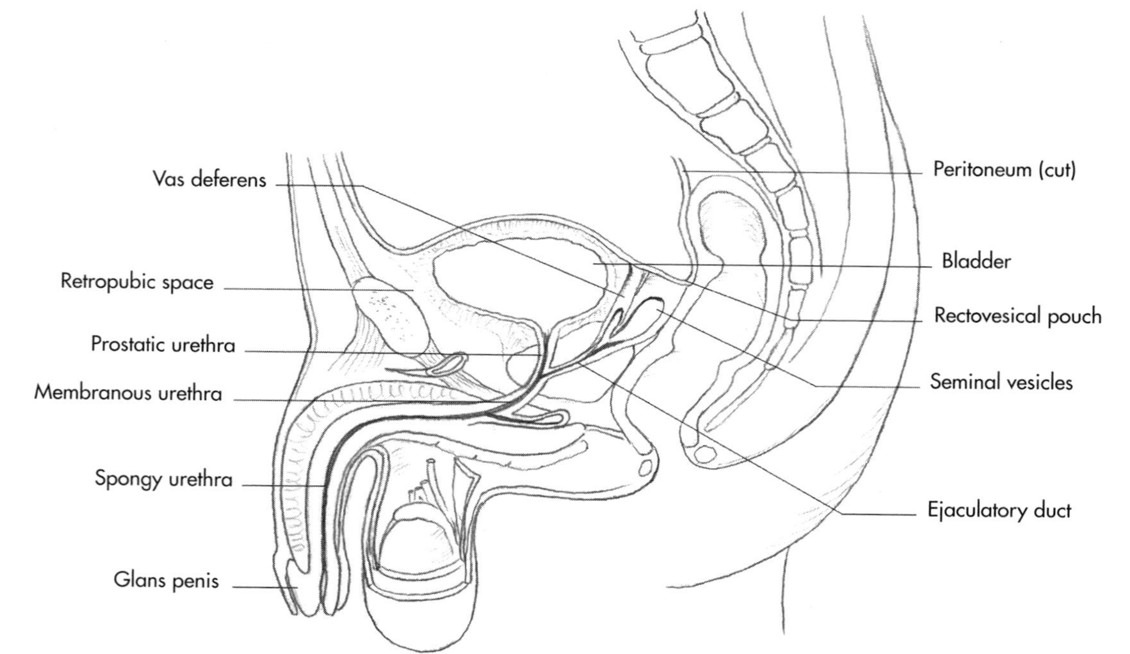

Figure 3.9 The male pelvis

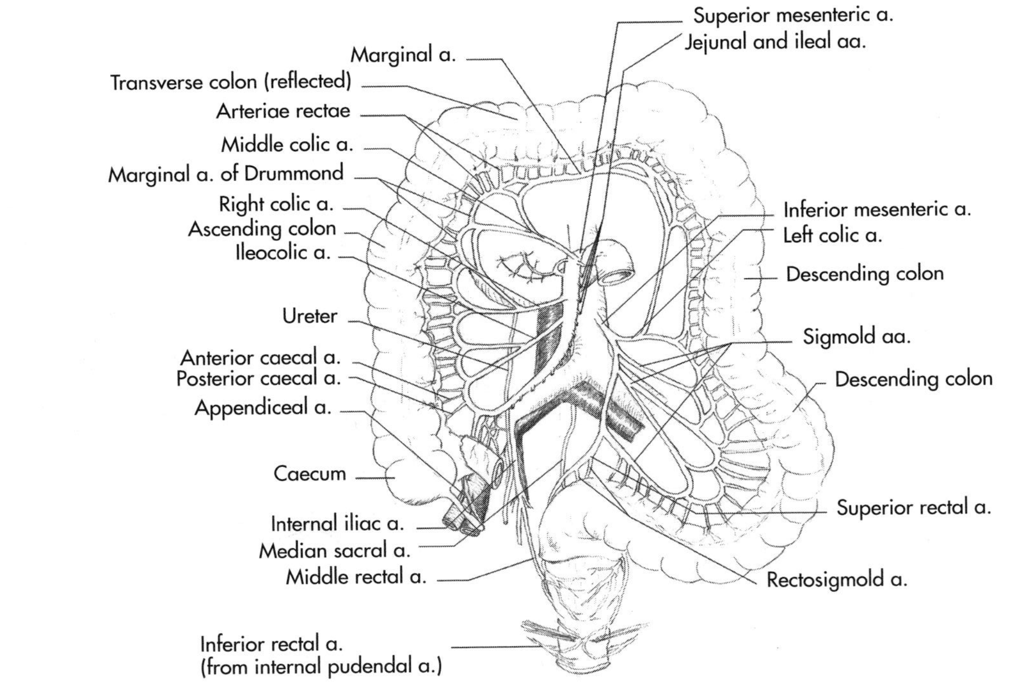

Superior mesenteric a.
Jejunal and ileal aa.
Marginal a.
Transverse colon (reflected)
Arteriae rectae
Middle colic a.
Marginal a. of Drummond
Right colic a.
Ascending colon
Ileocolic a.
Inferior mesenteric a.
Left colic a.
Descending colon
Ureter
Sigmold aa.
Anterior caecal a.
Posterior caecal a.
Descending colon
Appendiceal a.
Caecum
Superior rectal a.
Internal iliac a.
Median sacral a.
Middle rectal a.
Rectosigmold a.
Inferior rectal a.
(from internal pudendal a.)

Figure 3.10 Blood supply of the large intestine

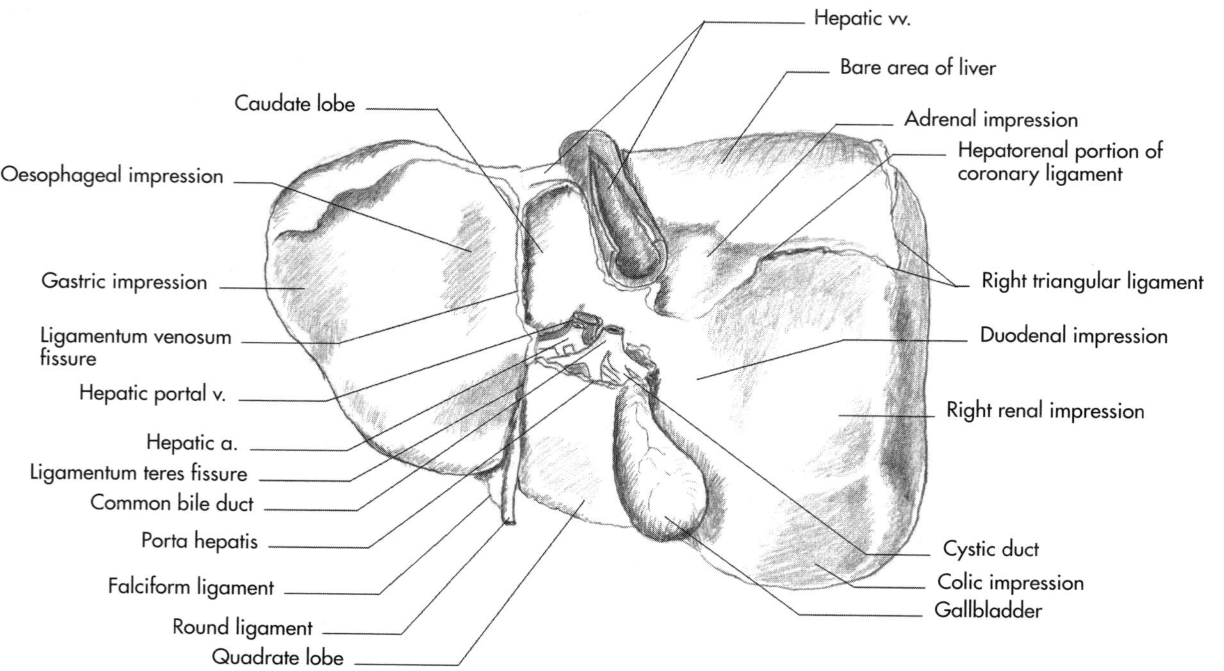

Figure 3.11 Liver, visceral surface

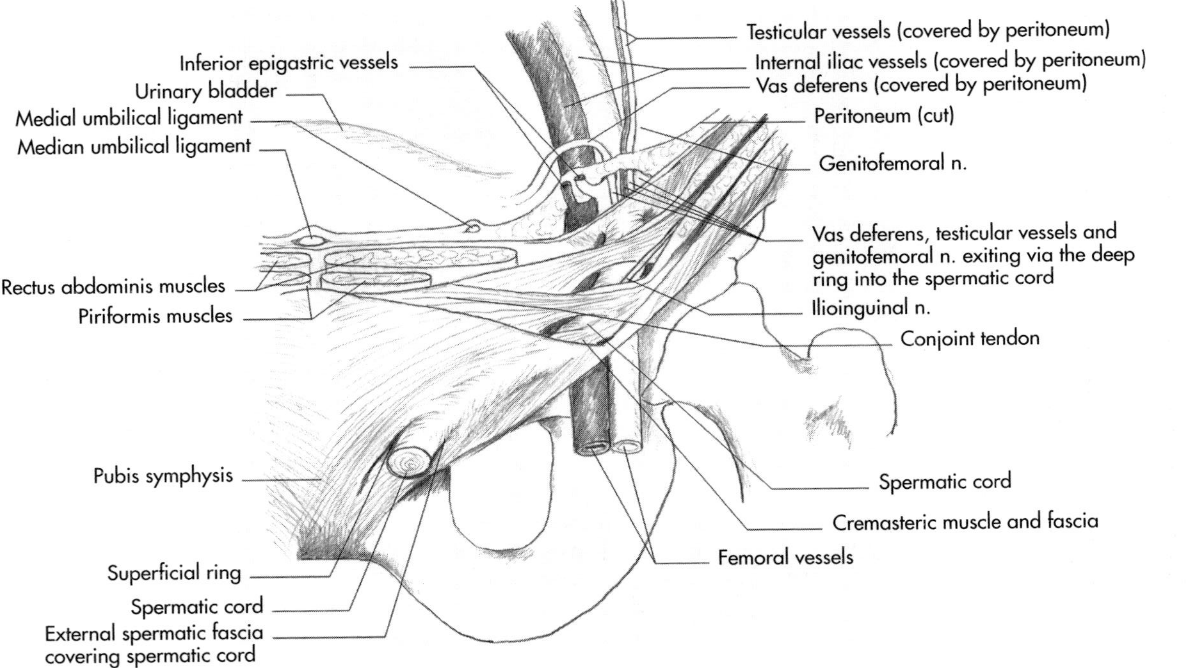

Figure 3.12 The male inguinal region showing the inguinal canal and spermatic cord

CHAPTER 4: MUSCULOSKELETAL SYSTEM

SKIN

What are the layers of the skin?

The skin consists of two main layers: the epidermis and dermis.

What are the properties of the epidermis?

It is essentially **avascular**.
Its function is **cornification**, which is creation of a tough layer of dead cells.

How thick is it?

It is 0.04–1.6 mm thick, depending on the site (thicker on the palms and soles, thinner on the eyelids).

What cells constitute the epidermis?

Epidermis contains four types of cells: keratinocytes, melanocytes, Langerhans' cells and Merkel's cells.

What are the properties of the dermis?

It contains the vascular bed of the skin and its function is **temperature regulation**. It also contains nerves and glandular elements of the skin.

How thick is it?

It is 15–40 times thicker than the epidermis. It can be divided into two layers: the **superficial papillary layer** and the **deep reticular layer**.

What are Langer's lines?

The alignment of collagen fibres in the dermis reveal patterns of lines over the body that allow folding of the skin. They are followed for surgical incisions.

What are the functions of skin?

Protects against:
- mechanical injury
- bacterial invasion
- ultraviolet light
- water.

Sensory for:
- pain
- light touch
- temperature.

Involved in:
vitamin D production.

What lies underneath the dermis?

Subcutaneous tissue and superficial fascia.

What are nails?

Firm plates of dead cells derived from the most superficial layer of the epidermis.

What are the superficial and deep fasciae?

Fasciae lie beneath the skin, holding various structures together. The fascial planes and spaces provide sites and direction of spread for infection.
The superficial fascia: the fat-containing subcutaneous tissue underlying the skin. It acts as an insulating layer. Deeper layers condense into sheets at the perineum and lower abdominal wall.
The deep fascia: wraps individual organs as sheets, or surrounds organs as loose material.

BONE

What is the structure of bone?

Periosteum: a connective tissue membrane surrounding the bone.
Compact/cortical bone: outer layer.
Trabecular/cancellous bone: inner layer.
Endosteum: inner surface is lined by a layer of flattened cells.
Medullary cavity: found in long bones – consists of yellow fatty marrow or red haematopoietic marrow.

What is endochondral ossification?

The cartilage is removed and replaced with bone; it occurs in the skeleton from the second month of intrauterine life.

Where does long bone growth occur?

From the physis. It occurs by endochondral ossification of the cartilage continually produced by the cells of the physis. When growth ceases, epiphyseal bone and metaphyseal bone fuse.

What is the blood supply of bone?

Partly from a nutrient artery, which penetrates through a nutrient foramen and via a vascular network in the periosteum. There is also an intramedullary component.

How are joints classified?

Fibrous: limited movement, e.g. sutures of the skull.
Cartilaginous: limited movement
- primary, e.g. first costosternal joint
- secondary, e.g. pubic symphysis.

Synovial: contain synovial fluid, e.g. knee.

What is articular cartilage?

The normal hyaline cartilage covering bony articular surfaces. It is avascular and derives its nourishment from synovial fluid.

What are the surface-palpable surface features of the back?

C7: vertebra prominens.
T7: inferior angle of scapula.
L4: crests of iliac bones – level of lumbar puncture.

What are the abnormal curvatures of the spine?

Scoliosis: lateral deviation in the coronal plane associated with rotation.
Kyphosis: increased posterior convexity in the sagittal plane.
Lordosis: increased anterior convexity in the sagittal plane.

How many vertebrae are there?

Cervical: 7.
Thoracic: 12.
Lumbar: 5.
Sacrum: 5 fused.
Coccygeal: 3–5 fused.

What are the parts of a thoracic vertebra?

Body.
Pedicles.
Superior and inferior articular processes.
Pars interarticularis.
Spinous and transverse processes.
Lamina.
Vertebral foramen for the passage of the spinal cord.
Intervertebral foramen for the passage of the spinal nerves.

What is spondylolysis?

Affects 3–7% of the general population, the incidence increasing to 23–62% in athletes, resulting in low back pain, mostly at L5. There is a defect in the pars interarticularis that connects the superior and inferior articular facets, thought to be caused by repeated microtrauma, although it can be congenital.

What is spondylolisthesis?

Where the body of one vertebra slips forwards over the one below it. This can again be congenital or acquired.

Which vertebra supports the skull?

Atlas. The atlas articulates inferiorly with the axis.

How do the atlas and axis articulate?

The axis projects the dens upwards behind the anterior arch of the atlas. It is held in place by the transverse ligament of the atlas. This is the point of rotation for the skull.

What is the difference between a ligament and a tendon?

Tendon: a fibrocellular structure attaching muscle to bone.
Ligament: a fibrocellular structure connecting two bones.

What is spina bifida?

Posterior spine elements (lamina, facets and spinous processes) fail to develop, allowing the contents of the spinal cord to prolapse through the defect.

What is ankylosing spondylitis?	A seronegative spondyloarthropathy where bodies of the vertebrae become fused together, giving the radiological picture of 'bamboo spine'. There is reduced spinal movement and subsequent kyphosis.
What lies between the vertebral bodies?	**Intervertebral discs:** they consist of an outer ring of fibrous tissue known as the annulus fibrosis and a soft inner core known as the nucleus pulposus. **Hyaline cartilage:** between the disc and vertebral body at the endplate.
What is the function of the intervertebral discs?	The differences in anterior and posterior depth contribute to the curvature of the spine. Allow rotation of vertebrae and absorb compressive forces. Degenerative changes in the disc can predispose to herniation of the nucleus pulposus, compressing the spinal cord and/or spinal roots.
What would cause a herniated intervertebral disc?	Occurs most commonly in the lumbosacral region. Heavy lifting with flexion and underlying degenerative changes can predispose to this.
What are the 'red flag' signs of spinal cord compression/cauda equina syndrome?	Reduced anal sphincter tone (per rectal examination). Loss of bladder and bowel control. Perianal/perineal sensory loss (saddle anaesthesia). Lower limb neurological signs, e.g. foot drop from motor weakness.
How are the vertebra joined together?	Bodies and discs: anterior and posterior longitudinal ligaments. Arches and processes: ligamentum flavum, interspinous and supraspinous ligaments.

What is the thoracolumbar fascia?

A fascia separating the deep erector spinae muscles from the superficial trapezius, latissimus dorsi, levator scapulae, rhomboid muscles and muscles of the thoracic wall.

What is the suboccipital triangle?

A region of the neck bounded by the following three muscles:

above and medially: rectus capitis posterior major

above and laterally: obliquus capitis superior

below and laterally: obliquus capitis inferior.

It is covered by a layer of dense fibrofatty tissue, situated beneath the semispinalis capitis. The floor is formed by the posterior occipito-atlantal membrane and the posterior arch of the atlas. In the deep groove on the upper surface of the posterior arch of the atlas are the vertebral artery and the first cervical or suboccipital nerve.

What is the ligamentum nuchae?

A triangular ligament extending from the external occipital protuberance to the spine of the seventh cervical vertebra. It becomes continuous with the supraspinous ligament.

What are the atlas and axis?

The atlas is the first cervical vertebra and articulates with the occipital bone and the axis below. The axis is the second cervical vertebra and articulates above with the atlas via the two facets of the dens.

What is the dens?

Otherwise known as the odontoid process, it is a superior protuberance fused to the body of the axis, articulating with the anterior arch of the atlas. It is enclosed in the transverse ligament of the atlas, cruciform ligaments, and alar and apical ligaments to the occipital bone.

Which joints allow movements of the head/neck?

Atlanto-occipital joint: flexion, extension and some lateral flexion.
Atlantoaxial joint: rotation.

Where does the spinal cord terminate?

At around L1–2. The terminal area is known as the conus medullaris.

What continues below this?

The **cauda equina** is the continuation of the lower lumbar and sacral nerves. Nerves continue to exit the vertebral foramina. Note that cauda equina = horse's tail (Latin).

What is the blood supply to the spinal cord?

A single anterior spinal artery (vertebral).
Two pairs of posterior spinal arteries (posterior inferior cerebellar branches).
Anterior and posterior radicular branches (vertebral, cervical, posterior intercostal and lumbar arteries).

What is a spinal tap?

Synonymous with a lumbar puncture, it is the removal of cerebrospinal fluid (CSF). As the spinal cord terminates at L1–2, the tap is carried out at L4 where the meninges are still present. CSF lies in the subarachnoid space, between the arachnoid and pial layers.

What structures will the needle pass through?

Skin.
Supraspinous ligament.
Interspinous ligament.
Ligamentum flavum.
Dura.
Arachnoid.

Why is the epidural space important?

The epidural space surrounds the outer meningeal dura layer and extends laterally along the course of the spinal nerve. When this space is infiltrated with local anaesthetic, only local and distal nerves are affected.

What is the sympathetic trunk?

It is a linking of sympathetic ganglia by nerves traversing from the skull to the coccyx (ganglion impar). The two trunks lie on either side of the vertebral column on the posterior abdominal wall. Within the ganglia the preganglionic sympathetic nerves synapse. They leave the ganglia as postganglionic sympathetic nerves.

What are the ganglia otherwise known as?

Paravertebral ganglia. They allow the sympathetic nerves to ascend or descend to target vessels and plexuses. Sympathetic nerves only originate from spinal roots T1–L2.

How are they arranged?

Cervical: three ganglia – superior, middle, inferior (stellate) ganglia.
Thorax: 12 ganglia – greater, lesser and least splanchnic nerves.
Lumbar: four ganglia – lumbar splanchnic nerves.
Sacral: four or five ganglia – sacral splanchnic nerves, ganglion impar.

SHOULDER

What are the similarities between the upper limb and the lower limb?

General arrangement of bones from proximal to distal is similar.
Same joint types (shoulder/hip = ball and socket; elbow/knee = hinge; wrist/ankle = plane, phalanges = hinge).
Compartmentalisation of muscles with a single nerve per compartment and one or two major functions of the compartment.

Nerves originate off a plexus (brachial/lumbosacral), with the largest nerve posterior (sciatic/radial).

What are the differences between the upper and lower limbs?

Rotation during development:
- **upper:** external 45°
- **lower:** internal 90°.

Elbow and knee flex in opposite directions.
Palm = anterior; sole = posterior.

What are the differences in function between the upper limb and the lower limb

See Table 4.1.

Table 4.1

Upper limb	Lower limb
Built for manipulation	Built for stability
Shoulder girdle = highly mobile	Hip = more stable
Pronation/supination of forearm	Reduced mobility
Hand = generalised for different movements	Foot = specialised for weight support

What does the pectoral girdle consist of?

The clavicle, scapula and proximal humerus with their respective joints: sternoclavicular, acromioclavicular and glenohumeral.

What is the function of the clavicle?

A rigid support – the doubly curved clavicle serves as a strut, keeping the limb away from the thorax so that the arm has maximum freedom of motion.
Cervicoaxillary canal (passageway between neck and arm) – the clavicle also forms one of the boundaries of the canal, affording protection to the neurovascular bundle supplying the upper limb.
Shock – it transmits shock from the upper limb to the axial skeleton.

What is the function of the scapula?

The scapula is suspended on the thoracic wall by muscle forming a 'functional joint' called the scapulothoracic joint. These muscles act to stabilise and/or actively move the scapula. Active movements of the scapula help increase the range of motion of the shoulder joint.

What constitutes the sternoclavicular joint?

A strong gliding and rotating synovial joint. The three ligaments that hold the joint are the anterior/posterior, interclavicular and costoclavicular.

What are the ligaments of the acromioclavicular joint?

Coracoclavicular: coracoid process to inferior clavicle.
Acromioclavicular: acromion to clavicle tip.
Coracoacromial: provides a roof for the joint.

What are the rotator cuff muscles and their function?

Supraspinatus.
Infraspinatus.
Teres minor.
Subscapularis.
Intracapsular tendon of biceps.
They hold the humeral head in the shallow glenoid fossa.

How does the glenohumeral joint function?

A synovial joint: the glenoid fossa articulates with the humeral head with the aid of the glenoid labrum, which deepens the joint.

What are the parts of the humerus?

Upper end:
- head articulates with the glenoid cavity
- greater and lesser tubercles.

Shaft:
- spiral groove posteriorly.

Lower end:
- capitellum (lateral) articulates with radius

trochlea (medial) articulates with ulna
medial and lateral epicondyles.

What are the important nerves related to the humerus?

Axillary nerve: winds around the neck.
Radial nerve: applied to the spiral groove.
Ulnar nerve: posterior to the medial epicondyle.

What two main movements are possible at the elbow joint?

Flexion/extension.
Pronation/supination.

What type of joint is the elbow joint?

There are actually three types of joints that make up the entire elbow joint:
humeroulnar joint (simple hinge joint)
humeroradial joint (arthroidal joint between humeral capitulum and radial head)
proximal radioulnar joint.

CUBITAL FOSSA

What is the cubital fossa?

It is a triangular area in front of the elbow and is bounded by:
medially: pronator teres
laterally: brachioradialis
base: imaginary line between the humeral epicondyles
floor: supinator muscle and brachialis
roof: skin, fascia and bicipital aponeurosis.

What are its contents?

From medial to lateral:
median nerve
brachial artery
biceps tendon
radial nerve.

WRIST

What are the structures felt anteriorly at the wrist?

From medial to lateral:
- flexor carpi ulnaris tendon
- ulnar artery
- flexor digitorum superficialis tendons
- palmaris longus (can be absent)
- flexor carpi radialis tendon
- radial artery
- brachialis tendon.

What are the bones of the wrist joint and how can they be remembered?

(*Mnemonic:* **S**ome **L**overs **T**ry **P**ositions **T**hat **T**hey **C**an't **H**andle [palms facing upwards, thumbs pointing laterally].)

First (proximal) row, lateral to medial:
- **S**caphoid
- **L**unate
- **T**riquetrum
- **P**isiform.

Second (distal) row, lateral to medial:
- **T**rapezium
- **T**rapezoid
- **C**apitate
- **H**amate.

What is the anatomical snuff box?

It is the space bounded by the tendons of abductor pollicis longus (ventrally), extensor pollicis brevis (ventrally) and extensor pollicis longus (dorsally).

What lies in the anatomical snuff box?

Radial artery.
Superficial branch of the radial nerve.
Scaphoid bone.

What is the flexor retinaculum?

It is a fibrous band that stretches across the concave anterior surface of the wrist, creating the carpal tunnel. The retinaculum is attached medially to the pisiform bone and the hook of the hamate and laterally to the tubercle of the scaphoid and a ridge on the trapezium.

What is carpal tunnel syndrome?

This is compression of the median nerve passing underneath the flexor retinaculum. This leads to paraesthesia and weakness of muscles in its distribution.

What are the causes of carpal tunnel syndrome?

Myxoedema.
O**E**dema (e.g. premenstrual).
Diabetes.
Idiopathic (most common).
Acromegaly.
Neoplasm.
Trauma.
Rheumatoid arthritis.
Amyloidosis.
Pregnancy.
(*Mnemomic*: MEDIAN TRAP.)

What is the extensor retinaculum?

It is a fibrous band that stretches across the dorsal surface of the wrist. It extends from the lateral border of the radius, spanning obliquely across the wrist to the triquetral and pisiform bones.

What function does it serve?

It holds down the long flexor and extensor tendons.

What are the structures passing superficial to the flexor retinaculum?

From medial to lateral:
- flexor carpi ulnaris tendon
- ulnar nerve
- ulnar artery
- palmar cutaneous branch of the ulnar nerve
- palmaris longus (can be absent).
- palmar cutaneous branch of median nerve.

What are the structures passing deep to the flexor retinaculum?

From medial to lateral:
- flexor digitorum superficialis tendons

flexor digitorum profundus tendons
median nerve
flexor pollicis longus
flexor carpi radialis tendon.

What are the structures passing superficial to the extensor retinaculum?

From medial to lateral:
- dorsal cutaneous branch of ulnar nerve
- basilic vein
- cephalic vein
- superficial branch of the radial nerve.

What are the structures passing deep to the extensor retinaculum?

From medial to lateral:
- extensor carpi ulnaris
- extensor digiti minimi
- extensor digitorum and extensor indicis
- extensor pollicis longus and extensor pollicis brevis
- extensor carpi radialis longus and extensor carpi radialis brevis
- abductor pollicis longus.

What is a ganglion?

A cystic swelling arising from the synovial lining of a joint or tendon. It is thought to be a myxomatous degeneration of fibrous tissue, although the exact cause is unknown. It is not attached to the overlying skin.

What is the palmar aponeurosis?

It is a triangular thickening of the deep fascia. It has an apex attached to the flexor retinaculum and its base divides into four slips that become attached to the flexor sheaths of the medial four fingers.

What is Dupuytren's contracture?

Fibrosis of the palmar aponeurosis, most commonly affecting the ring and little fingers. This leads to flexion of the metacarpophalangeal (MCP) and proximal interphalangeal (PIP) joints. There are several associations including:

Diabetes mellitus
Epilepsy
Age (positive correlation)
Family history (autosomal dominant)/**f**ibromatoses, e.g. Ledderhose's disease (fibrosis of the plantar aponeurosis)
Epileptic medication (e.g. phenobarbital)
Smoking
Trauma and heavy manual labour
Peyronie's disease of the penis
AIDS
Idiopathic
Liver disease (secondary to alcohol).

(*Mnemonic:* DEAFEST PAIL.)

What is Volkmann's contracture of the forearm?

Fibrosis of the flexor and extensor muscles of the forearm secondary to ischaemia (e.g. after supracondylar fracture with vascular compromise). This leads to flexion of the wrist, extension of MCP joints and flexion of the interphalangeal joints.

What is the pulp space?

It is the space filled with subcutaneous fat between fibrous septa overlying the palmar aspect of the distal phalanx.

Why is it important?

When infection occurs and pus collects, this leads to severe pain. The blood supply to the distal phalanx can thrombose, leading to ischaemia of the tip of the digit.

MEDIAN NERVE

What are the branches of the median nerve in the hand?

The median nerve divides into two in the palm, the lateral portion supplying the thenar muscles and sensation to the lateral three and a half digits, and the medial portion supplying the lateral two lumbricals and medial sensation.

The **palmar branch** arises at the lower forearm and pierces the carpal ligament. It then divides into lateral and medial branches in the hand, which supply sensation to the skin over the base of the thumb and the palm respectively.

What are the thenar muscles?

(*Mnemonic:* **LOAF**.)

Lateral two lumbricals.
Opponens pollicis.
Abductor pollicis brevis.
Flexor pollicis longus.

How is it examined?

Sensory: test sensation to the lateral three and a half digits (i.e. thumb, index, middle and lateral half of ring fingers, with palm facing upwards).

Motor: ask the patient to put their palm facing up and point their thumb in the air; tell them to keep it in that position while you try to push it down towards their palm (testing the autonomous nerve supply to the abductor policis brevis, the only muscle that the median nerve always supplies).

ULNAR NERVE

What are the branches of the ulnar nerve in the hand?

The ulnar nerve divides into a deep motor a and superficial sensory branch just beyond the **pisiform bone**. Its sensory supply is to the medial one and a half digits. Its motor supply is to the intrinsic muscles of the hand (medial two lumbricals and the interossei) and adductor pollicis.
Isolated sensory loss is possible with certain injuries.

How is it examined?

Sensory: test sensation to the medial one and a half digits (i.e. little finger and medial half of the ring, with the palm facing upwards).
Motor: ask the patient to hold a piece of paper between thumb and radial side of index finger while you try to pull it away using your thumb and index finger. If adductor pollicis is weak then compensation by flexor pollicis longus will lead to an excessively flexed posture of the thumb interphalangeal joint (**Froment's sign**). Test the dorsal interossei (autonomous supply) by asking the patient to spread his or her fingers against resistance.
(*Mnemonic:* PAD = **p**almar **i**nterossei **a**dduct and DAB = **d**orsal **i**nterossei **a**bduct.)

RADIAL NERVE

What are the branches of the radial nerve in the hand?

There are no major branches in the hand.

What does it supply?

Its sensory supply is to the extensor surface (dorsum) of the hand and forearm. Its motor supply is to the hand and finger extensors.

How is it tested?

Sensory: test sensation over the dorsum of the first web space.
Motor: ask patient to hold his hand out flat, palm down. Ask him or her to hold it straight while you push down on the fingers. This tests the MCP joint extensors (extensor digitorum communis, extensor digiti minimi and extensor indicis proprius), which are the autonomous muscles of the radial nerve.

LOWER LIMB

Which nerves supply the lower limb?

Lumbar and most of the sacral ventral rami of the lumbosacral plexus.
Superior and inferior gluteal (L5–S2): buttock and gluteal region.
Femoral (L2–4): anterior thigh, medial leg and extensors of the knee.
Obturator (L2–4): medial thigh and adductor muscles.
Sciatic (L4–S3): posterior part of the thigh and flexors of the knee.
Tibial (S1–2): posterior aspect of the leg and plantar aspect of the foot.
Common peroneal (L5–S2): anterior aspect of the leg and dorsum of the foot.

What is meralgia paraesthetica?

Entrapment of the lateral femoral cutaneous nerve of the thigh, leading to sensory symptoms on the anterolateral aspect of the thigh.

What is the blood supply of the lower limb?

See Figure 4.1.

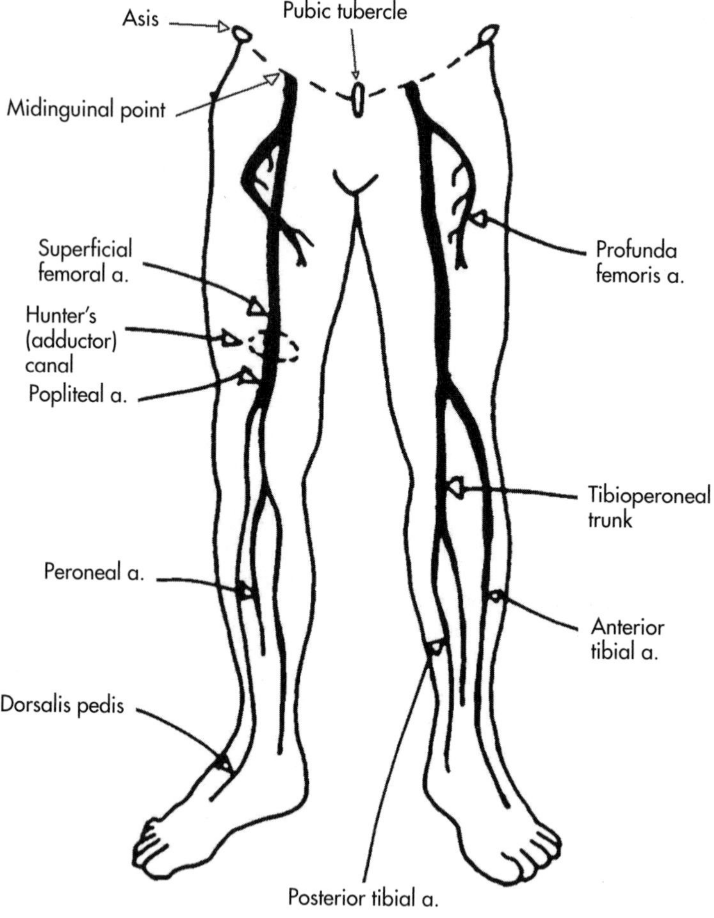

Figure 4.1

What is the landmark for the (common) femoral artery?

Midinguinal point (feel here for femoral pulse).

What are the branches of the common femoral artery?

After entering the thigh, it gives off four cutaneous arteries:

superficial circumflex iliac artery
superficial epigastric artery (an important landmark in the inguinal region!)
superficial external pudendal artery
deep external pudendal artery.

It then divides into:

profunda femoris artery (supplies the thigh muscles)
superficial femoral artery, which enters the adductor (Hunter's) canal.

What happens to the superficial femoral artery in the popliteal fossa?

It becomes the popliteal artery and then trifurcates into:

1. Anterior tibial artery.
2. Posterior tibial artery.
3. Peroneal artery.

What pulses are palpable in the foot?

The dorsalis pedis and the posterior tibial.

What are their landmarks?

Dorsalis pedis: at the dorsum of the foot between the extensor hallucis longus and extensor digitorum longus tendons (or the tendons of the big and second toes!).
Posterior tibial: midway along an imaginary line joining the point of the heel and the medial malleolus.

What are the venous tributaries of the lower limb?

See Figure 4.2.

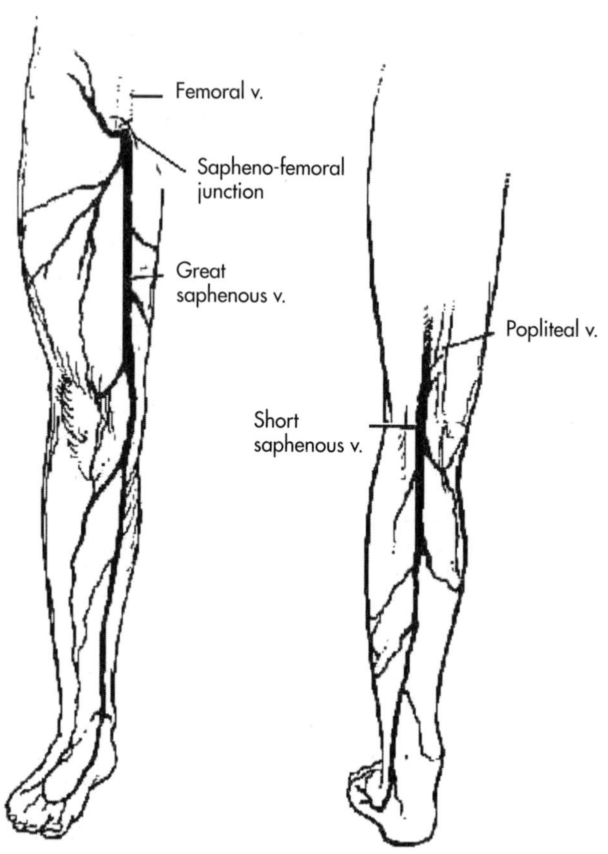

Figure 4.2

What is the course of the long saphenous vein?

Begins in front of the medial malleolus and travels upwards along the medial surface of tibia towards the knee. Passes one hand's-breadth medial to the patella and runs up the medial aspect of the thigh.

Enters the cribriform fascia 3.5 cm below and lateral to the pubic tubercle.

What is the course of the short saphenous vein?

Begins behind the lateral malleolus and runs upwards along the surface of the calf to drain into the popliteal vein at the level of the popliteal fossa.

What does the long saphenous vein drain into?

The femoral vein, after perforating the cribriform fascia at the saphenous opening, which is located inferior to the inguinal ligament and lateral to the pubic tubercle.

At what levels are its perforators?

Long saphenous vein: at 5, 10 and 15 cm above the medial malleolus, at Hunter's canal and at the saphenofemoral junction (SFJ).
Short saphenous vein: at the popliteal fossa.

What is the significance of these perforators?

They communicate with the deep venous system via a one-way valve system (blood drains from superficial to deep).

What happens if these valves become incompetent?

There is backflow of blood into the superficial system, i.e. varicose veins (see below).

Where is the SFJ?

Where the saphenous vein dives deep to join the femoral vein, medial to the femoral pulse, or 2 cm below and lateral to the pubic tubercle.

Which veins drain at the SFJ?

1. Superficial circumflex iliac vein.
2. Superficial epigastric vein.
3. Superficial external pudendal vein.
4. Deep external pudendal vein.

What are varicose veins?

Tortuous enlargements of the superficial veins of the lower limbs.

What is the Trendelenburg test for varicose veins?

Used to test the patency of the deep veins and is important when considering varicose vein surgery. Veins in the legs are drained by raising the limb. Then the SFJ is occluded by the hand or with a tourniquet. When the leg is lowered, rapid filling of the veins indicates that the perforating veins are incompetent and the blood is entering from the deep system. If rapid filling occurs only when pressure on the SFV is released, the incompetence lies at the junction.

Where does the lymph in the inguinal nodes drain from?

Buttock.
Abdominal wall.
Perineum.
External genitalia.
Lower part of anal canal and vagina.
Superficial tissues of leg and thigh.

What are the compartments of the thigh?

Extensor, flexor and adductor compartments. These are separated by the lateral, intermediate and medial intermuscular septa.

What is the intertrochanteric line?

Where the neck joins the shaft of the femur, the roughened ridge created anteriorly is called the intertrochanteric line. The intertrochanteric crest lies posteriorly.

What is the obturator canal?

An opening within the obturator membrane for the passage of the obturator vessels and nerve. Its boundaries are the edge of the obturator membrane, together with the obturator groove of the pubic bone. It is a rare site for hernias.

What is the femoral triangle?

It is a musculofascial triangle space on the anterior surface of the thigh.

Its boundaries are:
- **superior:** inguinal ligament
- **lateral:** medial border of sartorius
- **medial:** medial border of adductor longus
- **floor:** iliacus, tendon of psoas, pectineus and adductor longus (from lateral to medial)
- **roof:** the superficial cribriform fascia (containing lymph nodes and great saphenous vein)
- **contents:** femoral vein, artery, nerve (*Mnemonic:* VAN, from medial to lateral) and the deep inguinal lymph nodes. The profunda femoris is given off here.

What is the femoral sheath?

It is a downward prolongation of transversalis and iliacus fascia under the inguinal ligament.
Anterior wall: derived from fascia transversalis.
Posterior wall: derived from fascia iliaca (covering iliacus muscle).
Its divided by septa into three compartments:
- **medial:** femoral canal
- **intermediate:** conveys femoral vein
- **lateral:** conveys femoral artery.

Why is it important?

As it contains the femoral canal connecting the abdominal cavity to the lower limb, it is a potential site for a hernia.

What is the femoral canal?

The femoral canal is the medial compartment of the femoral sheath; it opens into the abdominal cavity superiorly at the **femoral ring**. It is about 1.5 cm in length.

Contents:
plug of fat
constant of Cloquet (lymph node of femoral canal).

Normal functions:
it gives space for the femoral vein to distend
lymphatic pathway.

Why is it important?

Site of development of femoral hernia. Within the ring, Cloquet's lymph node may become palpable, implying an underlying femoral hernia. A palpable node in this region is always a femoral hernia until proved otherwise.

What is the femoral ring?

The femoral ring is the superior opening into the femoral canal.
Its boundaries are:
medial: lacunar ligament (Gimbernat's ligament)
lateral: fascia on the femoral vein
anterior: inguinal ligament
posterior: pectineal ligament (Cooper's ligament).

Why is it important?

Its rigid boundaries can endanger the viability of the hernial contents.

What is the adductor (Hunter's/subsartorial) canal?

A musculofascial space that contains the neurovascular bundle of the anterior thigh. It begins proximally at the inferior angle of the femoral triangle and ends distally at the adductor hiatus.

What are its boundaries?

Anteromedial:
sartorius
aponeurotic fascia extending between vastus medialis and adductor longus and magnus.

	Anterolateral: vastus medialis. **Posterolateral:** adductor longus adductor magnus.
What are the contents of the adductor canal?	Femoral **A**rtery, and Its descending **G**eniculate branch. Femoral **V**ein. Long **S**aphenous nerve. **N**erve to vastus medialis. Deep **L**ymphatics. (*Mnemonic:* **A G**ood **V**alet **S**hould **N**ever **L**augh.)
What is the cruciate anastomosis?	The collateral circulation existing if the femoral artery is obstructed. The gluteal branches of the internal iliac anastomose with circumflex arteries, creating a path to the profunda femoris and femoral arteries.
What are the progressive symptoms of an obstructed artery?	Intermittent claudication. Rest pain. Ischaemia.
What are the symptoms of an acutely obstructed artery?	Six Ps: paraesthesia pallor pain perishingly cold (poikilothermia) pulseless paralysis.
What is the adductor hiatus?	A parting in the attachment of the adductor magnus to linea aspera. The femoral vessels become popliteal vessels at this point.
What structures pass through the greater sciatic foramen?	The structures are divided into those exiting above and below the piriformis muscle. The nerve to the obturator internus exits through the greater sciatic foramen and re-enters through the lesser sciatic foramen.

Below piriformis:
posterior femoral cutaneous nerve
nerve to quadratus femoris
inferior gluteal nerve and vessels
pudendal nerve
nerve to obturator internus (L5–S2)
sciatic nerve
internal pudendal vessels.

Above piriformis:
superior gluteal vessels
piriformis muscle.

What structures pass through the lesser sciatic foramen?

Nerve to obturator internus.
Tendon of obturator internus.
Pudendal vessels and nerve.

What is the hip joint?

A synovial ball-and-socket joint integrating the cartilage-covered spherical head of the femur and an incomplete ring of the cartilage lining the acetabulum. The depth of the socket is increased by the acetabular labrum (made of fibrocartilage).

Describe the fibrous capsule of the hip joint.

The proximal attachments are the margin of the acetabulum and the transverse acetabular ligament. Distally, it covers the head and neck of the femur, attaching close to the intertrochanteric line anteriorly. It does not reach the intertrochanteric crest posteriorly. It is reflected back over the neck, creating longitudinal folds called retinacula.

What ligaments reinforce the capsule?

Pubofemoral.
Ischiofemoral.
Iliofemoral.

What is the blood supply to the head of the femur?

Femoral branches: lateral and medial circumflex arteries.
Obturator branch: runs in the ligament of the head of the femur.

Nutrient artery: through substance of the bone.

What muscles are related to the hip?

Anterior:
pectineus
iliopsoas
rectus femoris.
Posterior:
piriformis
obturator internus
gemelli
quadratus femoris.
Superior:
gluteus minimus, medius and maximus.

What are the degenerative changes found in the hip in osteoarthritis?

Loss of joint space.
Osteophytes.
Subchondral sclerosis.
Subchondral cyst formation.
(*Mnemonic:* **LOSS**.)

How does this compare with osteoporosis?

In osteoporosis there is a reduction of bone mass per unit volume, predisposing the bone to fractures.

How are hip fractures classified anatomically?

Femoral head fracture: fracture involving the femoral head. This is usually the result of high-energy trauma.
Neck of femur fracture: also known as subcapital or intracapsular. Fracture proximal to the intertrochanteric line within the capsule. These fractures have a propensity to damage the blood supply to the femoral head, potentially leading to avascular necrosis.
Intertrochanteric fracture: fracture line between the greater and lesser trochanter on the intertrochanteric line.

Subtrochanteric: fracture involving the shaft of the femur immediately below the lesser trochanter; can extend down the shaft of the femur.

Name some causes of sciatic nerve injury.

Posterior dislocation of hip joint.
Penetrating injury (e.g. injection).
Iatrogenic (e.g. related to total hip arthroplasty).

What are the sequelae of a sciatic nerve injury?

Muscle paralysis: hamstrings and all the muscles of the leg and the foot.
Motor loss: all movements below the knee, with foot drop.
Sensory: complete below the knee except the medial side of the leg, foot and big toe, which is supplied by the saphenous branch of the femoral nerve.

What is the popliteal fossa?

It is a diamond-shaped anatomical area on the posterior aspect of the knee. It can be considered as a continuation of the adductor canal.

What are its boundaries?

Superomedial: tendons of semimembranosus and semitendinosus.
Superolateral: tendon of biceps femoris.
Inferomedial and inferolateral: medial and lateral heads of gastrocnemius.
Roof: the deep fascia (pierced by the short saphenous vein as it ends in the popliteal vein), superficial fascia, posterior femoral cutaneous nerve, skin.
Floor: from above, downwards:
- popliteal surface of the femur
- posterior aspect of knee joint
- popliteus muscle.

What are its contents?

From out inwards:
- tibial nerve (crosses from the lateral to medial side)
- popliteal vein
- popliteal artery.

The common peroneal nerve runs along the medial aspect of the biceps tendon.
Other contents are fat and popliteal lymph nodes.

What is the differential diagnosis for a popliteal mass?

Vascular masses:
- popliteal artery aneurysm (most common in popliteal fossa)
- cystic adventitial degeneration of popliteal artery.

Non-vascular masses:
- Baker's cyst
- popliteal cysts
- bursae (e.g. related to semimembranosus)
- soft tissue tumour:
  - benign: peripheral nerve sheath tumours
  - malignant: myxoid liposarcoma (adults), lipoblastoma (children)
- meniscal cyst
- traumatic tear of gastrocnemius.

What is a Baker's cyst?

Intrinsic intra-articular disorders cause joint effusion and swelling. The cyst protects the joint from potentially destructive pressures. The new sac is located outside the joint, posterior to the medial femoral condyle, between the tendons of the medial head of gastrocnemius and semimembranosus.

What are the condyles and epicondyles of the knee?

The condyles are found on the lower femur and upper tibia, both laterally and medially. They are expanded areas of bone that articulate with the knee joint. Both condyles bear epicondyles.

What is Osgood–Schlatter disease?

A self-limited knee condition in adolescent boys and girls characterised by pain and oedema of the tibial tubercle. During periods of rapid growth, stress from contraction of the quadriceps is transmitted through the patellar tendon onto the partially developed tibial tuberosity.

What are the ligaments of the knee?

Patellar ligament: a continuation of quadriceps to the tibial tuberosity.
Tibial collateral ligament: medial femoral epicondyle to medial shaft of tibia.
Fibular collateral ligament: lateral femoral epicondyle to head of fibula.
Oblique popliteal ligament: expansion of semitendinosus.
Cruciate ligaments: anterior and posterior, running from the intercondylar area to the lateral and medial femoral condyles.

Why can hip pain be referred to the knee?

The joint is innervated by branches of the sciatic, femoral and obturator nerves, all of which innervate the hip.

What are the bursae surrounding the knee joint?

Suprapatellar: used for joint aspiration.
Prepatellar: site of housemaid's knee.
Deep infrapatellar.
Subcutaneous infrapatellar: site of clergyman's knee.
Bursae associated with tendons and muscles:
- under semimembranosus
- under sartorius, gracilis and semitendinosus

under medial head of gastrocnemius (often into joint)
under lateral head of gastrocnemius (sometimes into joint)
under lateral collateral ligament
under popliteus (into joint).

What do the compartments of the leg contain?

Anterior:
tibialis anterior
extensor digitorum longus
extensor hallucis longus
fibularis tertius
deep peroneal nerve
tibial artery and vein.

Lateral:
fibularis longus
fibularis brevis
superficial peroneal nerve.

Deep posterior:
tibialis posterior
flexor digitorum longus
flexor hallucis longus
tibial nerve
posterior tibial artery
peroneal artery.

Superficial posterior:
gastrocnemius
plantaris
soleus.

What is the extensor retinaculum?

It is a continuation of the deep fascia thickened into bands holding down tendons that pass in relation to the ankle. These tendons are usually covered with synovium.

What are the structures passing anterior to the extensor retinaculum?

From medial to lateral:
saphenous nerve
great saphenous vein
superficial peroneal nerve.

What are the structures passing beneath or through the extensor retinaculum?

From medial to lateral:
- **T**ibialis anterior
- extensor **H**allucis longus
- anterior tibial **A**rtery and its **V**enae comitantes
- deep peroneal **N**erve
- extensor **D**igitorum longus
- **P**eroneus tertius.

(*Mnemonic:* **T**om **H**as **A** **V**ery **N**asty **D**irty **P**ill.)

What are the structures passing behind the medial malleolus beneath or through the flexor retinaculum?

From medial to lateral:
- **T**ibialis posterior
- flexor **D**igitorum longus
- posterior tibial **A**rtery and its **V**enae comitantes
- tibial **N**erve
- flexor **H**allucis longus.

(*Mnemonic:* **T**om, **D**ick **A**nd a **V**ery **N**ervous **H**arry.)

What are the structures passing behind the lateral malleolus superficial to the superior peroneal retinaculum?

From medial to lateral:
- short saphenous vein
- sural nerve.

What are the structures passing behind the lateral malleolus beneath or through the superior peroneal retinaculum?

Peroneus longus and brevis muscles.

What is innervation of the ankle jerk?

L5–S1. Elicited on the Achilles tendon.

Name some causes of common peroneal nerve injury.

Fractures of neck of fibula.
Pressure, e.g. by a tight plaster cast.

What are the sequelae of a common peroneal nerve injury?

Muscle paralysis: anterior and lateral lower leg compartments.
Motor: foot drop and inversion of the foot.

	Sensory: anterior and lateral aspects of leg and foot (the medial side is supplied by the saphenous branch of the femoral and so is not affected). **Deformity:** high-stepping gait.
What are the movements of the ankle joint?	Plantarflexion. Dorsiflexion. Inversion. Eversion.
What are the ligaments supporting the ankle joint?	**Medial (deltoid) ligament:** talar part navicular part calcaneal part. **Lateral ligament:** anterior talofibular calcaneofibular posterior talofibular.
What is the most common classification of ankle fractures?	**The Weber AO system:** Type A: fracture of the fibula is below the ankle joint, typically transverse. Type B: fracture of the fibula begins at the level of the ankle joint and typically extends proximally in spiral or short oblique fashion. Type C: fracture of the fibula is initiated above the ankle joint and is associated with ligamentous injuries.
What is the cutaneous innervation of the foot?	Branches of the **tibial nerve:** sural nerve calcaneal branch medial and lateral plantar nerves.
How many layers of muscles are there in the foot?	Four.
What forms the plantar arch?	Lateral plantar artery and the dorsalis pedis artery.

What is the plantar fascia and what is plantar fasciitis?

The **plantar fascia** originates on the medial tubercle of the calcaneus and fans out over the bottom of the foot to insert onto the proximal phalanges and the flexor tendon sheaths. It forms the longitudinal arch of the foot and functions as a shock absorber as well an arch support. **Plantar fasciitis** is a degenerative process with or without inflammatory changes, which can include fibroblastic proliferation of the fascia. It thought to be caused by repetitive microtrauma to the fascia.

Table 4.2 Deep muscles of the back

Muscle	Origin	Insertion	Action	Innervation
Erector spinae: comprises iliocostalis, longissimus and spinalis				
Iliocostalis – lumborum – thoracis – cervicis	Sacrum Lumbar vertebral spines Iliac crest	Ribs and cervical transverse processes	Extension of spine	Dorsal rami of spinal nn.
Longissimus – thoracis – cervicis – capitis	Sacrum Lumbar vertebral spines Iliac crest	Mastoid process	Extension of spine	Dorsal rami of spinal nn.
Spinalis – thoracis – cervicis – capitis	Spinous processes	Spinous processes	Extension of spine	Dorsal rami of spinal nn.
Transversospinalis: comprises semispinalis, multifidus and rotatores				
Semispinalis	Thoracic and cervical transverse processes	Higher thoracic and cervical spinous processes Superior and inferior nuchal lines	Extension of spine	Dorsal rami of spinal nn.
Multifidus	Sacrum Iliacs Transverse processes	Higher spinous processes	Extension of spine	Dorsal rami of spinal nn.
Rotatores	Transverse processes of thoracic vertebrae	Higher vertebrae and laminae	Extension of spine	Dorsal rami of spinal nn.
Interspinales	Spinous processes	Spinous processes	Extension of spine	Dorsal rami of spinal nn.
Intertransversarii	Cervical: anterior and posterior tubercles Thoracic: transverse processes	Cervical: anterior and posterior tubercles Thoracic: transverse processes	Extension of spine	Dorsal rami of spinal nn.

Table 4.3 Occipital triangle muscles

Muscle	Origin	Insertion	Action	Innervation
Splenius	Upper thoracic spines Ligamentum nuchae	Superior nuchal line Mastoid process	Rotation of head Lateral neck flexion	Dorsal cervical rami
Rectus capitis posterior minor	Posterior tubercle of atlas	Inferior nuchal line	Extend the head on the atlas Rotation of atlas on axis	First dorsal cervical n.
Rectus capitis posterior major	Bifid spine of axis	Inferior nuchal line, lateral to minor muscle	Extend the head on the atlas Rotation of atlas on axis	First dorsal cervical n.
Obliquus capitis inferior	Bifid spine of axis	Transverse process of atlas	Extend the head on the atlas Rotation of atlas on axis	First dorsal cervical n.
Obliquus capitis superior	Transverse process of atlas	Between superior and inferior nuchal lines	Extend the head on the atlas Rotation of atlas on axis	First dorsal cervical n.

Table 4.4 Shoulder muscles

Muscle	Origin	Insertion	Action	Innervation
Trapezius	Superior nuchal line Nuchal ligament Spines of seventh and all thoracic vertebrae	Lateral third of clavicle Median margin of acromion Scapular spine	Elevates shoulder Laterally rotates scapula Retracts scapula on thoracic wall	Spinal accessory n.
Latissimus dorsi	Spinous processes of lower six thoracic vertebrae Lumbodorsal fascia Crest of ilium	Floor of intertubercular groove of humerus	Adducts, Extends, Medially rotates arm	Thoracodorsal n.
Levator scapulae	Transverse processes of C1–4	Medial border of scapula above root of scapular spine	Raises scapula	Dorsal scapular n.
Rhomboid minor	Spine of seventh cervical and first thoracic vertebrae lower part of nuchal ligament	Medial margin of scapula at the root of the scapular spine	Retracts, Medially rotates scapula	Dorsal scapular n.
Rhomboid major	Spinous processes of second to fifth thoracic vertebrae	Medial border of scapula below root of scapular spine	Retracts, Medially rotates scapula	Dorsal scapular n.

Table 4.4 Shoulder muscles (continued)

Muscle	Origin	Insertion	Action	Innervation
Supraspinatus[a]	Supraspinous fossa of scapula	Superior aspect of greater tuberosity of humerus	Abducts the arm (first 15°)	Suprascapular n.
Infraspinatus[a]	Infraspinous fossa of scapula	Midportion of greater tuberosity of humerus	Laterally rotates the arm	Suprascapular n.
Teres minor[a]	Lateral border of scapula	Lower aspect of greater tuberosity of humerus	Laterally rotates arm	Axillary n.
Teres major	Inferior medial border of scapula	Crest of lesser tuberosity of humerus	Adducts, Medially rotates arm	Lower subscapular n.
Deltoid	Lateral third of clavicle Acromion process Scapular spine	Deltoid tuberosity of humerus	Abduction of arm from 15° to 90°	Axillary n.
Subscapularis[a]	Subscapular fossa (anterior surface of scapula)	Lesser tuberosity of the humerus	Medially rotates the arm	Upper and lower subscapular nn.
Triceps, long head	Infraglenoid tubercle of scapula	Olecranon process of ulna	Extends arm and forearm	Radial n.

[a] Rotator cuff: supraspinatus, infraspinatus, teres minor and subscapularis stabilise the shoulder joint through their insertion into the humeral head.

Table 4.5 Pectoral region muscles

Muscle	Origin	Insertion	Action	Innervation
Pectoralis major	Medial half of the clavicle Manubrium and body of sternum Costal cartilages of ribs 2–6	Lateral lip of bicipital groove	Flexes, adducts, medially rotates the arm	Medial and lateral pectoral nn.
Pectoralis minor	Ribs 3–5	Coracoid process of the scapula	Draws the scapula forwards and downwards	Medial pectoral n.
Subclavius	First rib and its cartilage	Inferior surface of the clavicle	Depresses the clavicle	Nerve to subclavius
Serratus anterior[a]	Ribs 1–8	Medial border of the scapula on its costal (deep) surface	Draws the scapula forwards The inferior fibres rotate the scapula superiorly	Long thoracic n.

[a] Paralysis of serratus anterior (as a result of injury to its nerve, e.g. during breast surgery) leads to winging of the scapula.

Table 4.6 Arm muscles

Muscle	Origin	Insertion	Action	Innervation
Anterior compartment				
Biceps brachii	Short head: tip of the coracoid process of the scapula Long head: supraglenoid tubercle of the scapula	Tuberosity of the radius	Flexes the elbow Supinates the forearm Flexes shoulder (long head)	Musculocutaneous n.
Brachialis	Anterior surface of the lower half of the humerus and the associated intermuscular septa	Coronoid process of the ulna	Flexes the forearm	Musculocutaneous n.
Coracobrachialis	Coracoid process of the scapula	Medial side of the humerus at midshaft	Flexes, Adducts the arm	Musculocutaneous n.
Posterior compartment				
Triceps brachii	Long head: infraglenoid tubercle of the scapula Lateral head: upper part of the posterior surface of humerus Medial head: lower part of the posterior surface of humerus	Olecranon process of the ulna	Extends the forearm The long head extends and adducts arm	Radial n.

Table 4.7 Forearm muscles

Muscle	Origin	Insertion	Action	Innervation
Anterior superficial compartment[a]				
Pronator teres	Medial epicondyle of humerus Coronoid process of ulna	Lateral aspect of shaft of radius	Pronates hand Flexes forearm	Median n.
Flexor carpi radialis	Medial epicondyle of humerus	Bases of second and third metacarpal bones	Flexes forearm and hand Aids in pronation and abduction of hand	Median n.
Palmaris longus	Medial epicondyle of humerus	Flexor retinaculum and palmar aponeurosis	Flexes hand	Median n.
Flexor digitorum superficialis	Humeroulnar head: medial epicondyle of humerus and coronoid process of ulna Radial head: oblique line on anterior border of radius	Tendons split to attach to lateral sides of middle phalanges	Flexes phalanges, wrist and forearm	Median n.
Flexor carpi ulnaris	Humeral head: medial epicondyle of humerus Ulnar head: olecranon process and posterior border of ulna	Pisiform Hook of hamate Base of fifth metacarpal	Flexes forearm and hand Adducts hand	Ulnar n.
Anterior deep compartment				
Flexor pollicis longus	Radius and adjacent interosseous membrane	Base of distal phalanx of thumb	Flexes thumb	Anterior interosseous n. (branch of median n.)

Table 4.7 Forearm muscles (continued)

Muscle	Origin	Insertion	Action	Innervation
Flexor digitorum profundus	Upper three-quarters of anterior aspect of ulna and adjacent interosseous membrane	Base of distal phalanges of fingers	Flexes phalanges	Radial half by anterior interosseous n. Ulnar half by ulnar n.
Pronator quadratus	Distal anterior aspect of ulna	Distal anterior aspect of radius	Pronates hand	Anterior interosseous n.
Lateral compartment				
Brachioradialis	Upper two-thirds of the lateral supracondylar ridge of the humerus	Lateral side of the base of the styloid process of the radius	Flexes the elbow, assists in pronation and supination	Radial n.
Extensor carpi radialis longus	Lower third of the lateral supracondylar ridge of the humerus	Dorsum of the second metacarpal bone (base)	Extends the wrist Abducts the hand	Radial n.
Posterior compartment				
Extensor carpi radialis brevis	Lateral epicondyle of humerus (common extensor origin)	Dorsum of the third metacarpal bone (base)	Extends the wrist Abducts the wrist	Deep branch of radial n.
Extensor digitorum	Lateral epicondyle of humerus	Extensor expansion (middle and distal phalanges) of medial four fingers	Extends the fingers (DIP, PIP and MCP joints) Extends wrist	Deep branch of radial n.

Table 4.7 Continued

Muscle	Origin	Insertion	Action	Innervation
Extensor digiti minimi	Lateral epicondyle of humerus	Extensor expansion of the fifth digit	Extends the DIP, PIP and MCP joints of the fifth digit	Deep branch of radial n.
Extensor carpi ulnaris	Lateral epicondyle of humerus	Medial side of the base of the fifth metacarpal	Extends the wrist; adducts the hand	Deep branch of radial n.
Anconeus	Lateral epicondyle of the humerus	Lateral side of the olecranon and the upper quarter of the ulna	Extends the forearm	Deep branch of radial n.
Supinator	Lateral epicondyle of humerus Annular ligament Ulna	Upper half of anterior surface of radius and its lateral surface	Supinates the forearm (following pronation)	Deep branch of radial n.
Abductor pollicis longus	Middle third of the posterior surface of the radius and ulna	Base of the first metacarpal	Abducts the thumb at carpometacarpal joint	Deep branch of radial n.
Extensor pollicis brevis	Distal part of posterior surface of the radius	Base of the proximal phalanx of the thumb	Extends the thumb at the MCP joint	Deep branch of radial n.
Extensor pollicis longus	Middle part of the posterior surface of the ulna	Base of the distal phalanx of the thumb	Extends the thumb at the IP joint	Deep branch of radial n.
Extensor indicis	Distal part of posterior surface of the ulna	Extensor expansion of index	Extends the MCP joint of the index finger	Deep branch of radial n.

DIP, distal interphalangeal; IP, interphalangeal; MCP, metacarpophalangeal; PIP, proximal interphalangeal.

[a] All muscles of this group are supplied by the median nerve and its branches except flexor carpi ulnaris and medial half of flexor digitorum profundus.

Table 4.8 Hand muscles

Muscle	Origin	Insertion	Action	Innervation
Small muscles of the hand				
Palmaris brevis	Flexor retinaculum, palmar aponeurosis	Skin of the palm near the ulnar border of the hand	Draws the skin of the ulnar side of the hand towards the centre of the palm	Superficial branch of the ulnar n.
Palmar interossei (4)[a]	First arises from base of the first metacarpal; remaining three muscles arise from the palmar surface of the shafts of second, fourth and fifth metacarpals	Proximal phalanges and extensor expansion of first, second, fourth and fifth fingers	Adduction of the digits towards the third digit (PAD)	Ulnar nerve, deep branch
Dorsal interossei (4)[a]	Four muscles, each arising from two adjacent metacarpal shafts	Proximal phalanges and the extensor expansion of the second, third, fourth and fifth digits	Abduction of digits from the third digit (DAB)	Ulnar n., deep branch
Lumbricals (4)	Tendons of flexor digitorum profundus (digits 2–5)	Extensor expansion of medial four digits	Flex the MCP joints Extend the proximal and DIP joints	Median n. (radial 2) via palmar digital nn. and ulnar n. (ulnar 2) via deep branch
Short muscles of the thumb				
Adductor pollicis	Oblique head: capitate, second and third (base) metacarpals Transverse head: third metacarpal (shaft)	Base of the proximal phalanx of the thumb	Adducts the thumb	Ulnar n., deep branch

Table 4.8 Continued

Muscle	Origin	Insertion	Action	Innervation
Abductor pollicis brevis	Flexor retinaculum Scaphoid Trapezium	Base of the proximal phalanx of thumb	Abducts thumb	Median n.
Flexor pollicis brevis	Trapezium and flexor retinaculum	Proximal phalanx of the thumb	Flexes the carpometacarpal and MCP joints of the thumb	Median n.
Opponens pollicis	Trapezium and flexor retinaculum	Shaft of first metacarpal bone	Opposes the thumb	Median n.
Short muscles of the little finger				
Abductor digiti minimi (hand)	Pisiform	Base of the proximal phalanx of the little finger	Abducts the little finger	Deep branch of the ulnar n.
Flexor digiti minimi brevis (hand)	Hook of hamate and flexor retinaculum	Proximal phalanx of the little finger	Flexes the little finger	Ulnar n., deep branch
Opponens digiti minimi	Hook of hamate and flexor retinaculum	Medial border of fifth metacarpal bone	Opposes the little finger	Ulnar n., deep branch

[a] Both palmar and dorsal interossei flex the MCP joint and extend the PIP and DIP joints.

Table 4.9 Thigh muscles

Muscle	Origin	Insertion	Action	Innervation
Anterior compartment				
Sartorius	Anterosuperior iliac spine	Upper medial surface of tibial shaft	Flexes, abducts, laterally rotates hip Flexes and medially rotates the knee	Femoral n. (L2–3)
Iliacus	Iliac fossa	Lesser trochanter of femur	Flexes hip If thigh is fixed, it flexes the trunk on the thigh as in sitting up	Femoral n. (L2–3)
Psoas major	Transverse processes, bodies and intervertebral discs of 12 thoracic and five lumbar vertebrae	Lesser trochanter of femur	Same as iliacus	Lumbar plexus (L1–3)
Pectineus	Superior ramus of pubis	Upper end shaft of femur	Flexes and adducts hip	Femoral n. (L2–3)
Quadriceps femoris (anterior compartment) which consists of the following four muscles:				
Rectus femoris	Straight head: anteroinferior iliac spine Reflected head: ilium above the acetabulum	Into patella and then through ligamentum patellae into tibial tubercle	Extension of knee	Femoral n. (L2–4)
Vastus lateralis	Upper end and shaft of femur	Quadriceps tendon into patella	Extension of knee	Femoral n. (L2–4)
Vastus medialis	Upper end and shaft of femur	Quadriceps tendon into patella	Extension of knee	Femoral n. (L2–4)
Vastus intermedius	Shaft of femur	Quadriceps tendon into patella	Extension of knee	Femoral n. (L2–4)

Table 4.[illegible] Continued

Muscle	Origin	Insertion	Action	Innervation
Medial compartment				
Gracilis	Inferior ramus of pubis Ramus of ischium	Medial surface of upper part of shaft of tibia	Adducts hip Flexes knee	Obturator n. (L2–3)
Adductor longus	Body of pubis	Posterior surface of shaft of femur	Adducts hip Assists in lateral rotation	Obturator n. (L2–4)
Adductor brevis	Inferior ramus of pubis	Posterior surface of shaft of femur	Adducts hip Assists in lateral rotation	Obturator n. (L2–4)
Adductor magnus	Inferior ramus of pubis Ischial ramus Ischial tuberosity	Posterior surface of shaft of femur Adductor tubercle of femur	Adducts hip Assists in lateral rotation of hip Hamstring part: extends thigh	Adductor portion: obturator n. Hamstring part: tibial part of sciatic n. (L2–4)
Obturator externus	Outer surface of obturator membrane	Trochanter fossa of femur	Lateral rotator of hip	Obturator n. (L3–4)
Posterior compartment				
Biceps femoris (short head)	Shaft of femur	Head of fibula	Flexes and laterally rotates knee	Common peroneal part of sciatic n.
Biceps femoris (long head)	Ischial tuberosity	Head of fibula	Flexes and laterally rotates leg Extends thigh	Tibial part of sciatic n.
Semitendinosus	Ischial tuberosity	Medial surface of upper part of tibia	Flexes and medially rotates leg Extends thigh	Tibial part of sciatic n.
Semimembranosus	Ischial tuberosity	Medial condyle of tibia	Flexes and medially rotates leg Extends thigh	Tibial part of sciatic n.
Adductor magnus (hamstring part)	Ischial tuberosity	Adductor tubercle of femur	Extends thigh	Tibial part of sciatic n.

Table 4.10 Leg muscles

Muscle	Origin	Insertion	Action	Innervation
Anterior compartment				
Tibialis anterior	Shaft of tibia and interosseous membrane	Medial cuneiform and base of first metatarsal	Extends the foot at ankle Inverts foot at subtalar and transverse tarsal joints Helps to maintain the medial longitudinal arch of the foot	Deep peroneal n. (L4–5)
Extensor digitorum longus	Anterior shaft of fibula	Extensor expansion of lateral four toes	Extends toes Dorsiflexes foot	Deep peroneal n. (L5, S1)
Peroneus tertius	Anterior shaft of fibula	Base of fifth metatarsal	Dorsiflexes foot Everts foot at subtalar and transverse tarsal joints	Deep peroneal n. (L5, S1)
Extensor hallucis longus	Anterior shaft of fibula	Base of distal phalanx of big toe	Extends big toe Dorsiflexes foot Inverts foot at subtalar and transverse tarsal joints	Deep peroneal n. (L5, S1)
Extensor digitorum brevis	Calcaneus	Long extensor tendons to second, third and fourth toes	Extends toes	Deep peroneal n. (S1,2)
Extensor hallucis brevis	Calcaneus	Proximal phalanx of big toe	Extends big toe	Deep peroneal n.

Table 4.10 Continued

Muscle	Origin	Insertion	Action	Innervation
Lateral compartment				
Peroneus longus	Shaft of fibula (lateral surface)	Base of first metatarsal Medial cuneiform	Plantarflexes foot (at ankle) Everts foot at subtalar and transverse tarsal joints Supports lateral longitudinal arch and transverse arch of the foot	Superficial peroneal n. (L5, S1–2)
Peroneus brevis	Shaft of fibula (lateral surface)	Base of fifth metatarsal	Plantarflexes foot Everts foot at subtalar and transverse tarsal joints Holds up lateral longitudinal arch	Superficial peroneal n. (L5, S1–2)
Posterior compartment (superficial and deep)				
Superficial group				
Gastrocnemius	Medial and lateral condyles of femur	Calcaneum (via tendo calcaneum)	Plantarflexes foot Flexes knee	Tibial n. (S1–2)
Plantaris	Lateral supracondylar ridge of femur	Calcaneum	Plantarflexes foot Flexes knee	Tibial n. (S1–2)
Soleus	Shafts of tibia and fibula	Calcaneum (via tendo calcaneum)	With gastrocnemius, a powerful plantarflexor of ankle (walking and running)	Tibial n. (S1–2)

Table 4.10 Leg muscles (continued)

Muscle	Origin	Insertion	Action	Innervation
Deep group				
Popliteus	Lateral condyle of the femur	Posterior surface of the tibia above soleal line	Flexes the knee Unlocks the knee	Tibial n. (L4–5, S1)
Tibialis posterior	Shafts of tibia and fibula and interosseous membrane	Tuberosity of navicular bone	Plantarflexes foot Inverts foot at subtalar and transverse tarsal joints Supports medial longitudinal arch of the foot	Tibial n. (L4–5)
Flexor digitorum longus	Shaft of tibia	Bases of distal phalanges of lateral four toes	Flexes distal phalanges of lateral four toes Plantarflexes foot Supports lateral longitudinal arch of foot	Tibial n. (S2–3)
Flexor hallucis longus	Shaft of fibula	Base of distal phalanx of big toe	Flexes distal phalanx of big toe Plantarflexes foot Supports medial longitudinal arch of the foot	Tibial n. (S2–3)

Table 4.11 Foot muscles

Muscle	Origin	Insertion	Action	Innervation
First layer				
Abductor hallucis	Medial tubercle of calcaneum	Base of proximal phalanx of the big toe	Flexes big toe Abducts big toe Supports medial longitudinal arch	Medial plantar n. (S2–3)
Flexor digitorum brevis	Medial tubercle of calcaneum	Middle phalanges of four lateral toes (perforated by those of flexor digitorum longus)	Flexes lateral four toes Supports medial and lateral longitudinal arches	Medial plantar n. (S2–3)
Abductor digiti minimi	Medial and lateral tubercles of calcaneum	Base of proximal phalanx of fifth toe	Flexes fifth toe Abducts fifth toe Supports lateral longitudinal arch	Lateral plantar n. (S2–3)
Second layer				
Accessory flexor (quadratus plantae)	Medial and lateral sides of calcaneum	Tendon flexor digitorum longus	Aids flexor digitorum longus in flexing lateral four toes	Lateral plantar n. (S2–3)
Lumbricals (4)	Tendons of flexor digitorum longus	Dorsal extensor expansion of lateral four toes	Extends toes at interphalangeal joints	First lumbrical: medial plantar Remainder: lateral plantar (S2–3)
Flexor digitorum longus tendons				
Flexor hallucis longus tendons				
Third layer				
Flexor hallucis brevis	Cuboid Lateral cuneiform Tibialis posterior insertion	Medial and lateral sides of base of proximal phalanx of big toe (by two tendons)	Flexes MTP joint of the big toe Supports medial longitudinal arch	Medial plantar n. (S2–3)

Table 4.11 Foot muscles (continued

Muscle	Origin	Insertion	Action	Innervation
Adductor hallucis, oblique head Transverse head	Bases of second, third and fourth metatarsals Heads of third, fourth and fifth metatarsals	Lateral side base proximal phalanx big toe	Adducts big toe Supports transverse arch (oblique head)	Deep branch lateral plantar n. (S2–3)
Flexor digiti minimi brevis	Base of fifth metatarsal	Lateral side base of proximal phalanx small toe	Flexes the MTP joint of little toe	Lateral plantar n. (S2–3)
Fourth layer				
Dorsal interossei (4)	Adjacent sides of metatarsals	Bases of phalanges and dorsal expansion of corresponding toes	Abduct toes (second toe as reference) Flex MTP joints Extend interphalangeal joints	Lateral plantar n. (S2–3)
Plantar interossei (3)	Third, fourth and fifth metatarsals	Bases of proximal phalanges of third, fourth and fifth toes	Adduct toes (second toe as reference) Flex MTP joints Extend interphalangeal joints	Lateral plantar n. (S2–3)
Peroneus longus tendon				
Tibialis posterior tendon				
Dorsum of foot				
Extensor digitorum brevis	Calcaneus	Long extensor tendons to second, third and fourth toes	Extends toes	Deep peroneal n. (S1–2)
Extensor hallucis brevis	Calcaneus	Proximal phalanx of big tow	Extends big toe	Deep peroneal n. (S1–2)

MTP, metatarsophalangeal.

Table 4.12 Upper limb arteries

Artery	Origin	Relations	Termination	Branches	Supply
Axillary a.[a]	At the lateral border of the first rib as a continuation of the subclavian a.	**The brachial plexus:** its cords have different relations according to their names, ie medial, lateral and posterior (no anterior cord) **Medial:** axillary vein	At lower border of the teres major muscle by becoming the brachial a.	**First part (one branch):** Superior thoracic a. **Second part (two branches):** Acromiothoracic a Lateral thoracic a. **Third part (three branches):** Subscapular a. Anterior humeral circumflex a. Posterior humeral circumflex a.	Supplies various structures via its branches
Brachial a.	As the continuation of the axillary a. at the distal edge of the teres major muscle	**Medial:** related to the ulnar n. and basilic vein. It is superficial along its course being covered by fascia and skin only **Anterior:** median n. and biceps m. Crossed from lateral to medial by the median n. (at the level of midhumerus). Bicipital aponeurosis. Fascia and skin **Posterior:** triceps, insertion of coracobrachialis, brachialis and radial n.	In the cubital fossa at the level of the radial neck by dividing into radial and ulnar aa.	Profunda brachii (deep brachial) accompanies the radial n. Superior ulnar collateral a. Inferior ulnar collateral a. Terminal bifurcation to the radial a. and ulnar a.	Radial head Other structures via its branches

Table 4.12 Upper limb arteries (continued)

Artery	Origin	Relations	Termination	Branches	Supply
Radial a.	In the cubital fossa at the level of the radial neck from the bifurcation of the brachial a.	**Three parts:** Cubital fossa to apex of radial styloid Apex of radial styloid to proximal end of first metacarpal space on dorsum of hand From first metacarpal space to radial side of fifth metacarpal base – in palm of hand mainly as deep arch **Anterior:** its upper half is overlapped by brachioradialis distally lying between the tendons of brachioradialis and flexor carpi radialis, where it is covered by skin and fascia only **Posterior:** it is superficial to all muscles attached to the radius. It does not enter the carpal tunnel **Lateral:** in the middle third of the forearm it lies medial to the radial n.	Forms the deep palmar arch, anastomosing with the deep branch of ulnar a. on the radial side of the fifth metacarpal	**Forearm:** Radial recurrent a. Muscular branches Anterior radial carpal Superficial palmar a. arch **Dorsum of hand:** Posterior radial carpal Dorsalis pollicis Dorsalis indicis **Palm:** Princeps pollicis Radialis indicis Deep arch	Forearm and hand

Table 4.12 Continued

Artery	Origin	Relations	Termination	Branches	Supply
Ulnar a.	In the cubital fossa at the level of the radial neck from the bifurcation of the brachial a.	**Anterior:** flexor digitorum superficialis, pronator teres (both heads), flexor carpi radialis, palmaris longus, flexor carpi ulnaris, crossed by median n. **Posterior:** brachialis, flexor digitorum profundus. In its distal part it lies between the tendons of flexor carpi ulnaris and flexor digitorum superficialis and superficial to the carpal tunnel	On the radial side of the pisiform bone with bifurcation into superficial and deep branches. These anastomose with the radial a. branches' namesakes	**Forearm:** Anterior ulnar recurrent a. Posterior ulnar recurrent a. Common interosseous, quickly dividing to anterior and posterior interosseous aa. **Hand and palm:** Deep palmar a. arch Superficial palmar a. arch	

[a] Critical knowledge about the axillary artery:

Three parts:

The first part is between the lateral border of the first rib and the medial border of pectoralis minor.

The second part is behind pectoralis minor.

The third part is between the lateral border of pectoralis minor the inferior border of teres major.

Surgical importance:

Endangered during axillary dissection.

The most common site for aneurysms in the upper limb.

Table 4.13 Upper limb veins

Vein	Origin	Relations	Termination	Tributaries
Axillary v.[a]	At lower border of the teres major muscle as a continuation of the basilic vein joined with vena comitantes of the brachial a.	**Lateral:** Axillary a. and brachial plexus **Medially:** Pectoralis minor	At the lateral border of the first rib, where it becomes the subclavian v.	Cephalic and basilic vv. (laterally and medially, respectively) and tributaries corresponding to axillary a. branches

[a] It is arranged into superficial and deep systems.

Superficial system (more important):

Begins as an irregular venous network on the dorsum of the hand. The cephalic v. (laterally) and basilic v. (medially) migrate anteriorly, communicate via the median cubital v. and penetrate the deep fascia separately. The median antebrachial v. contributes.

Deep system:

Formed from the venae comitantes of the main arteries.

Table 4.14 Lower limb arteries

Artery	Origin	Relations	Termination	Branches	Supply
Femoral a.[a]	Continuation of the external iliac at the distal border of the inguinal ligament	It traverses the femoral triangle to its apex, accompanied by the femoral vein on its medial side. Enters the adductor canal, now the vein becomes posterior to it Exits the canal through the adductor hiatus to become the popliteal a.	At the opening in the adductor magnus by becoming the popliteal a.	**Superficial:** Superficial epigastric Superficial circumflex External pudendal **Deep:** Deep external pudendal Profunda femoris	Various structures via its branches
Profunda femoris a.	4 cm distal to the inguinal ligament as a branch of the femoral a.	Passes laterally and deeply, leaving the femoral triangle at the floor between pectineus and adductor longus **Anterior:** Adductor longus Femoral vein **Posterior:** Iliacus Pectineus Adductor magnus	Perforating the adductor magnus as the fourth perforating a.	Lateral circumflex Medial circumflex Muscular Perforating arteries	Various structures via its branches

Table 4.14 Lower limb arteries (continued)

Artery	Origin	Relations	Termination	Branches	Supply
Superficial epigastric and superficial circumflex aa.	Femoral a.	Superior epigastric arises from the front of the femoral artery about 1 cm below the inguinal ligament and, passing through the femoral sheath and the fascia cribrosa, turns upwards in front of the inguinal ligament and ascends between the two layers of the superficial fascia of the abdominal wall, almost as far as the umbilicus Superior circumflex pierces the fascia lata, runs laterally, parallel with the inguinal ligament, as far as the crest of the ilium	Anterior abdominal wall, anterosuperior iliac spine and the external genitalia	–	Inguinal region, anterior abdominal wall, subinguinal lymph nodes
Deep external pudendal a.	Femoral a.	Runs medially across pectineus and adductor longus deep to the facia lata. It pierces the fascia to supply the perineum	Perineum	–	Scrotum, labia majorum, perineum

Table 4.14 Continued

Artery	Origin	Relations	Termination	Branches	Supply
Medial and lateral circumflex aa.	Profunda femoris a.	Given off in the femoral triangle **Medial:** leave the floor between psoas major and pectineus, winding around the femur posteriorly **Lateral:** pass deep to sartorius and rectus femoris	Gluteus and hip	**Medial:** Ascending br. (anastomoses with inferior gluteal a.) Transverse br. (anastomoses with corresponding br. of lateral circumflex a.) **Lateral:** Ascending br. (hip joint and anastomoses with gluteal aa.) Transverse br. (anastomoses with corresponding br. of medial circumflex a.) Descending br. (anastomoses with genicular aa.)	Gluteal muscles and hip joint

Table 4.14 Lower limb arteries (continued)

Artery	Origin	Relations	Termination	Branches	Supply
Superior gluteal a.	Posterior trunk of internal iliac a.	Appears at the upper border of the piriformis m. running between gluteus medius and minimus	Anastomosis with circumflex and inferior gluteal aa. (cruciate anastomosis)	Muscular	Gluteus maximus, piriformis and tensor fascia lata
Inferior gluteal a.	Branch of anterior trunk of internal iliac a.	Appears at the lower border of the piriformis	Anastomosis with circumflex and inferior gluteal aa. (cruciate anastomosis)	–	Gluteus medius and minimus
Popliteal a.	As continuation of the femoral a. at the opening in the adductor magnus	**Superficial:** Fascia Posterior femoral cutaneous n. Short saphenous v. Popliteal v. **Deep:** Femur Popliteus and its fascia	At the distal edge of popliteus by division into anterior and posterior tibial a.	Anterior and posterior tibial Geniculate branches: two superior, middle, two inferior Muscular and cutaneous branches	Knee joint and various thigh and calf muscles through its branches

Table 4.14 Continued

Artery	Origin	Relations	Termination	Branches	Supply
Posterior tibial a.	At the distal border of popliteus from the bifurcation of popliteal a. into anterior and posterior tibial aa.	**Superficial:** Tibialis posterior Fascia and flexor retinaculum Gastrocnemius Soleus Tibial nerve Abductor hallucis brevis **Deep:** Skin Flexor digitorum longus Tibia (distal end)	At the distal border of the flexor retinaculum of the ankle by subdivision into medial and lateral plantar aa.	Circumflex fibular Peroneal Muscular Cutaneous Nutrient to tibia Medial and lateral plantar aa.	Posterior compartment leg muscles through its various branches
Medial plantar a.	At the distal medial border of flexor retinaculum from the bifurcation of posterior tibial a.		By joining the plantar digital artery from the lateral plantar artery to the medial side of the great toe	Digital, cutaneous and muscular	Digital, cutaneous and muscular, metatarsals
Lateral plantar a.	At the distal medial border of the flexor retinaculum from the bifurcation of the posterior tibial a.		At the plantar arch at the base of the first metatarsal by joining with dorsalis pedis	Muscular, medial calcaneal, cutaneous, plantar and dorsal metatarsal arteries and digital to little toe	Digital, cutaneous, muscular, metatarsals and calcaneus

Table 4.14 Lower limb arteries (continued)

Artery	Origin	Relations	Termination	Branches	Supply
Anterior tibial a.	At the distal border of the popliteus from the bifurcation of the popliteal a.	**Anterior:** Tibialis anterior Fascia Extensor retinaculum Extensor hallucis longus Extensor digitorum longus Anterior tibial nerve Skin **Posterior:** Front of ankle joint Interosseous membrane Front of tibia **Lateral:** Extensor hallucis longus Anterior tibial nerve Extensor digitorum longus	At the distal border of the ankle joint by changing its name to dorsalis pedis	Anterior tibial recurrent Posterior tibial recurrent Circumflex fibular Muscular Cutaneous Malleolar (lateral, medial)	Anterior compartment of the leg

Table 4.14 Continued

Artery	Origin	Relations	Termination	Branches	Supply
Dorsalis pedis a.	At the distal border of the ankle joint by continuation of the anterior tibial a.		On plantar aspect of the first metatarsal by joining lateral plantar a., forming the plantar arch	First metatarsal (dorsal, plantar) Arcuate artery Cutaneous Tarsal, medial and lateral	Dorsal surface of the foot
Peroneal a.	Branch of the posterior tibial a. shortly after its formation	Descends in the posterior compartment close to the fibula between tibialis posterior and flexor hallucis longus	At calcaneus	Muscular to posterior and lateral compartments Calcaneal Lateral malleolar Perforating branch to anterior tibial a.	Lateral compartment of leg

[a] It is now common to call the femoral a. above the origin of profunda femoris the 'common femoral a.' and to call it the 'superficial femoral a.' below it.

Table 4.15 Lower limb veins

Vein	Origin	Relations	Termination	Tributaries
Popliteal v.	Lower border of popliteus by the joining of anterior and posterior tibal vv.	Initially medial in the popliteal fossa, passes superficially to end posterolaterally to the popliteal a. Continues to pass through the adductor hiatus	As it passes through the adductor canal top, becomes the femoral v.	Small saphenous vein Anterior and posterior tibial Geniculate branches Muscular and cutaneous

Table 4.16 Lower limb nerves

Nerve	Source	Course and relations	Branches	Type
Femoral n.	L2–4 ventral rami	Appears at the lateral border of psoas, continuing between it and ilacus towards the inguinal ligament. It passes beneath the inguinal ligament lateral to the femoral a. As it enters the femoral triangle it has a very short course before dividing into anterior and posterior divisions	**From femoral nerve:** Nerve to iliacus Vasomotor to femoral artery **From anterior division:** Nerve to pectineus Medial cutaneous Intermediate cutaneous Nerve to sartorius **From posterior division:** Nerve to quadriceps femoris Saphenous nerve	**Motor:** Sartorius Pectineus Rectus femoris Vastus lateralis Vastus intermedius Vastus medialis
Saphenous n.	Cutaneous division of femoral n.	Descends in the adductor canal with the femoral vessels. It does not pass through the adductor canal but continues below the knee on the medial side of the leg to the medial aspect of the foot	–	**Sensory:** Medial aspect of lower leg and foot

Table 4.16 Lower limb nerves (continued)

Nerve	Source	Course and relations	Branches	Type
Superior gluteal n.	L4–S1	Appears at the upper border of piriformis running between gluteus medius and minimus	Muscular	**Motor:** Gluteus medius and minimus Tensor fascia lata
Inferior gluteal n.	L5–S2	Appears at the lower border of the piriformis m.	Muscular	**Motor:** Gluteus maximus
Obturator n.	L2–4 ventral rami	Divides into anterior and posterior divisions before passing with the obturator a. through the obturator canal	**Anterior division:** Articular to sacroiliac joint Articular to hip Pectineus Adductor longus and brevis To subsartorial plexus Vasomotor to femoral artery **Posterior division:** Obturator externus Adductor magnus	**Motor:** Adductor longus Adductor brevis Adductor magnus (adductor part) Gracilis Obturator externus **Sensory:** Skin of the lower medial thigh

Table 4.16 Continued

Nerve	Source	Course and relations	Branches	Type
Sacral and coccygeal plexus	**One nerve comes from five roots:** Sciatic (L4–S3) **Four nerves come from two roots:** Nerve to quadratus femoris Nerve to piriformis Nervi erigentes Nerves to anal muscles: coccygeus, levator ani, external sphincter **Six nerves come from three roots:** Superior gluteal Inferior gluteal Nerve to obturator internus Posterior femoral cutaneous Pudendal Sacrococcygeal			
Posterior femoral cutaneous n.	S1–3	Appears below piriformis, usually on the superficial aspect of the sciatic n. It descends in the thigh just beneath the fascia lata and pierces it at the popliteal fossa	Inferior cluneal branches	**Sensory:** Buttocks External genitalia Back of thigh Popliteal fossa Upper calf

Table 4.16 Lower limb nerves (continued)

Nerve	Source	Course and relations	Branches	Type
Sciatic n.	L4–S3 within the pelvis	Leaves the pelvis through the greater sciatic foramen. It usually terminates at the upper apex of the popliteal fossa by bifurcation into tibial and common peroneal nn. **Relations outside the pelvis** **Superficial:** Gluteus maximus Piriformis Long head of biceps **Deep:** Acetabulum Nerve to quadratus femoris Gemelli Obturator internus Quadratus femoris Obturator externus Adductor magnus **Medial:** Tuber ischii Semimembranosus Semitendinosus **Lateral:** Greater trochanter Gluteus maximus Short head of biceps femoris	Articular to hip joint Adductor magnus Semimembranosus Biceps femoris Semitendinosus	**Motor:** Semitendinosus Semimembranosus Biceps femoris Adductor magnus m. (hamstring part)

Table 4.16 Continued

Nerve	Source	Course and relations	Branches	Type
Common peroneal n.	At the bifurcation of the sciatic nerve, usually in the popliteal fossa. It terminates as the bifurcation of deep and superficial peroneal nn.	In the popliteal fossa it lies under cover of the laterally placed biceps femoris m. It winds around the lateral side of the head of the fibula in the substance of peroneus longus where it divides into its terminal branches	Lateral sural cutaneous n. and communicating branch (to the medial sural cutaneous n.) Geniculate lateral (superior and inferior) Deep peroneal Superficial peroneal Lateral cutaneous n. of calf	**Motor:** Gastrocnemius Plantaris Popliteus Soleus **Sensory:** Lateral side of the leg (sural communicating)
Superficial peroneal n.	From the bifurcation of the common popliteal in the substance of peroneus longus	It continues in the lateral compartment and terminates at the distal border of the extensor retinaculum by subdivision into medial and lateral branches, becoming cutaneous in the lower part of the leg. It runs between peroneus longus and peroneus brevis	–	**Motor:** Peroneus brevis, peroneus longus **Sensory:** Dorsum of foot except first digital cleft, distal third of leg
Deep peroneal n.	From the bifurcation of the common popliteal n. in the substance of peroneus longus	It pierces extensor digitorum longus and descends with anterior tibial vessels over the interosseous membrane, then over the ankle joint to lie between the tendons of tibialis anterior medially and extensor hallucis longus laterally	–	**Motor:** Tibialis anterior Extensor hallucis longus Extensor digitorum (longus and brevis) Peroneus tertius **Sensory:** First digital cleft

Table 4.16 Lower limb nerves (continued)

Nerve	Source	Course and relations	Branches	Type
Tibial n.	As a division of the sciatic n. with the common peroneal n.	It is the larger of the two terminal branches of the sciatic n. traversing the popliteal fossa superficial to the popliteal v. and a. It descends deep to the soleus m. accompanied by the posterior tibial vessels passing behind the medial malleolus, to end in medial and lateral planter nn. It terminates in medial and lateral plantars at the distal third of the flexor retinaculum	Medial sural cutaneous n. becoming sural n. (on receiving the communicating branch from the common peroneal n.) Calcaneal branches Plantar branches	**Motor:** Gastrocnemius Soleus Tibialis posterior Flexor hallucis longus Flexor digitorum longus **Sensory:** Articular to ankle and sole of foot Medial calcaneal Medial and lateral plantar
Medial plantar n. (L4–5)	Division from tibial n. at the flexor retinaculum	Accompanies the medial plantar a. towards the sole Between the first and second layers of the foot	–	**Motor:** Flexor digitorum brevis Flexor hallucis brevis First lumbrical **Sensory:** Plantar aspect of three and a half medial toes and the nail bed of these toes

Table 4.16 Continued

Nerve	Source	Course and relations	Branches	Type
Lateral plantar n. (S1–2)	Division from tibial n. at the flexor retinaculum	Accompanies the lateral plantar a. towards the sole Between the first and second layers of the foot	–	**Motor:** Abductor digiti minimi Flexor digiti minimi brevis Adductor hallucis brevis Lateral three lumbricals All interossei **Sensory:** Plantar aspect of one and a half medial toes and the nail bed of these toes.
Sural n.	Continuation of the medial sural cutaneous br. of the tibial n. after being joined by the communicating br. of the common peroneal n.	Follows the short saphenous v. distally and superficially appears from behind the lateral malleolus	–	**Sensory:** Calf Lateral side of foot Little toe

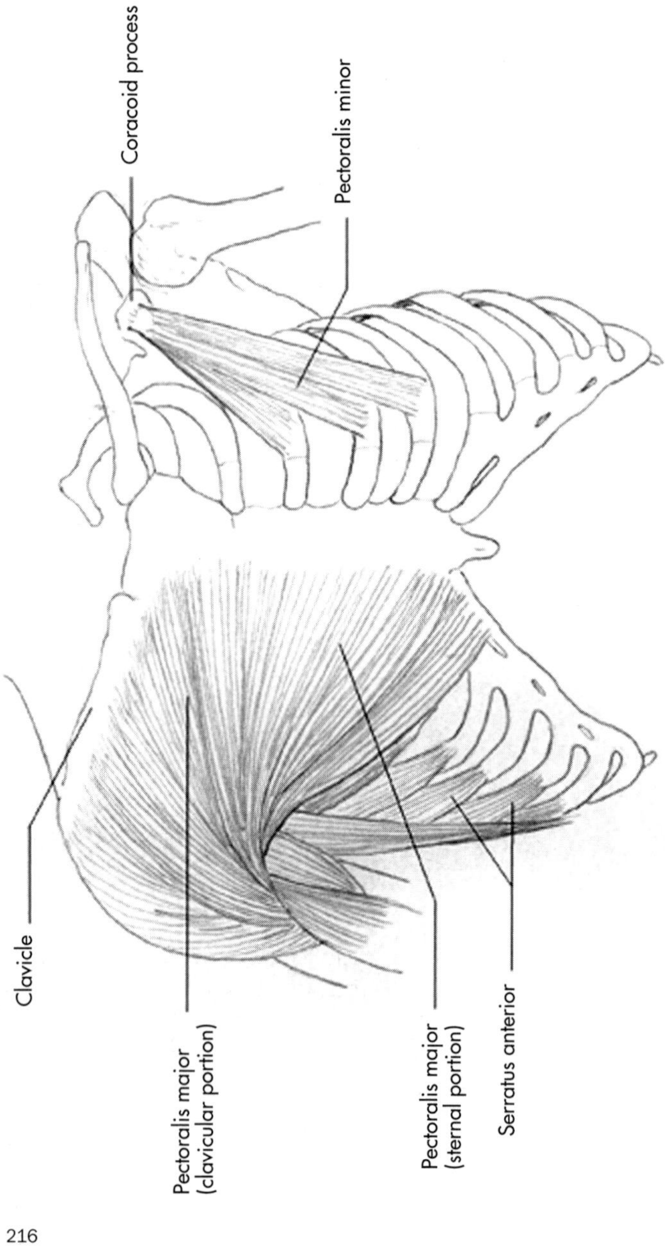

Figure 4.3 The pectoral muscles

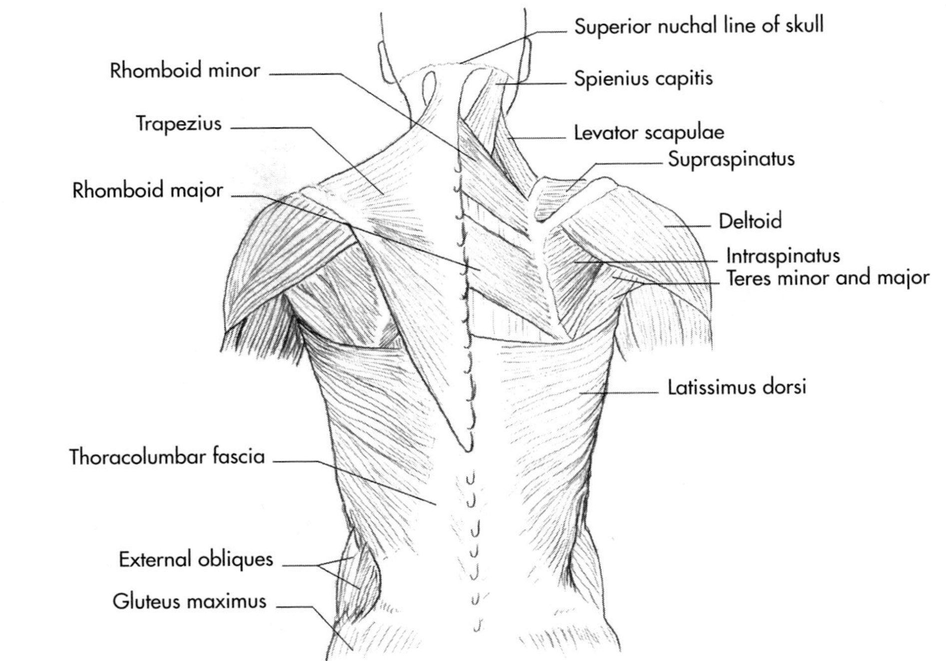

Superior nuchal line of skull
Rhomboid minor
Spienius capitis
Trapezius
Levator scapulae
Supraspinatus
Rhomboid major
Deltoid
Intraspinatus
Teres minor and major
Latissimus dorsi
Thoracolumbar fascia
External obliques
Gluteus maximus

Figure 4.4 Back muscles

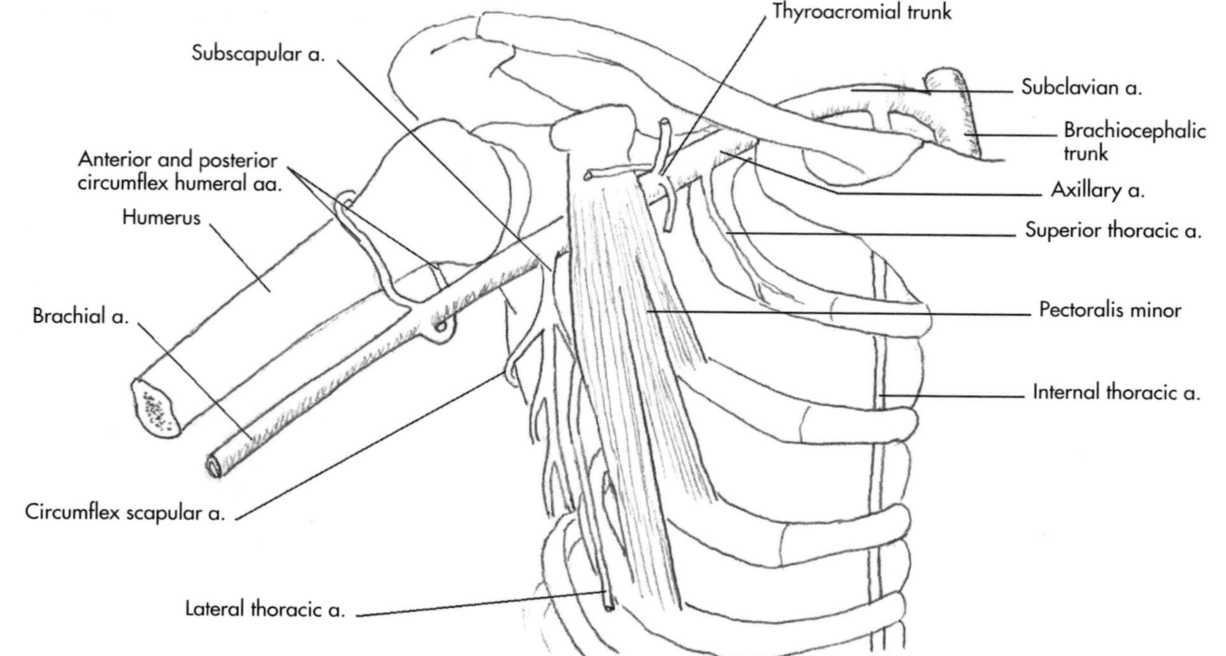

Figure 4.5 The axilliary artery and its branches

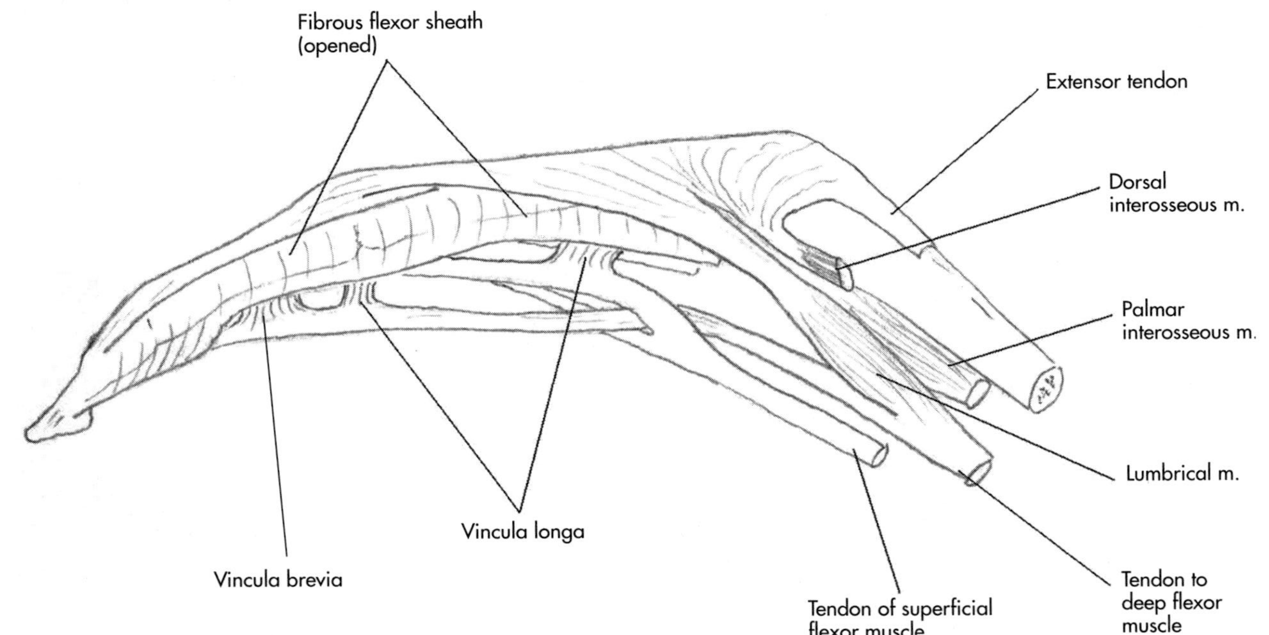

Figure 4.6 Dissection of the finger

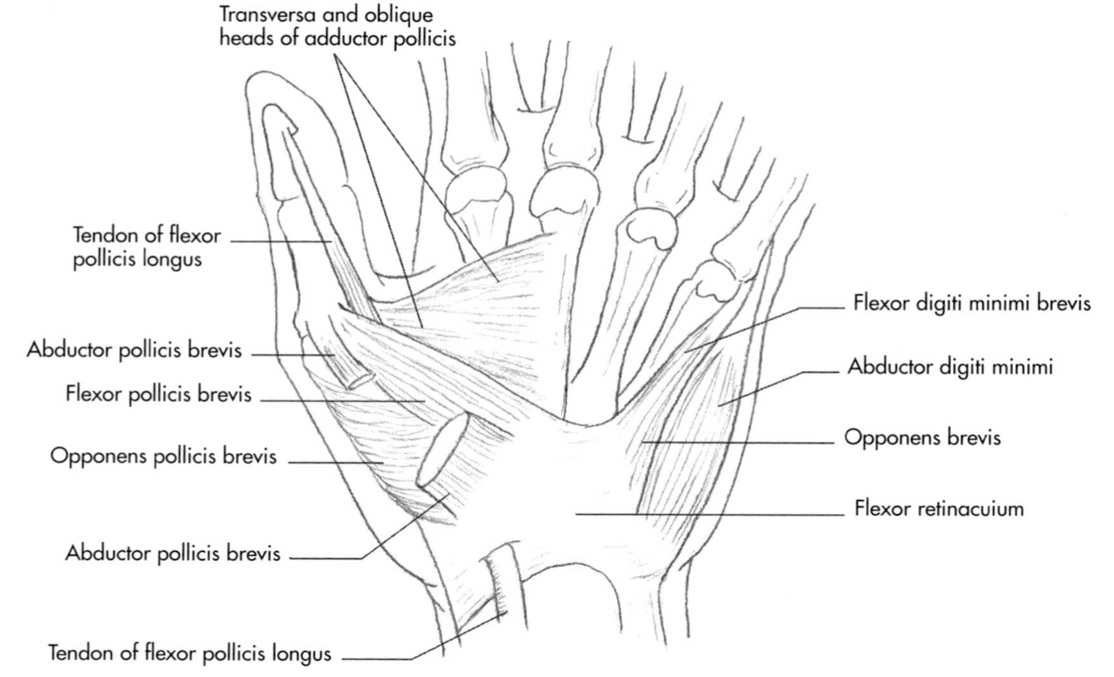

Figure 4.7 Thenar and hypothenar muscles of the palm

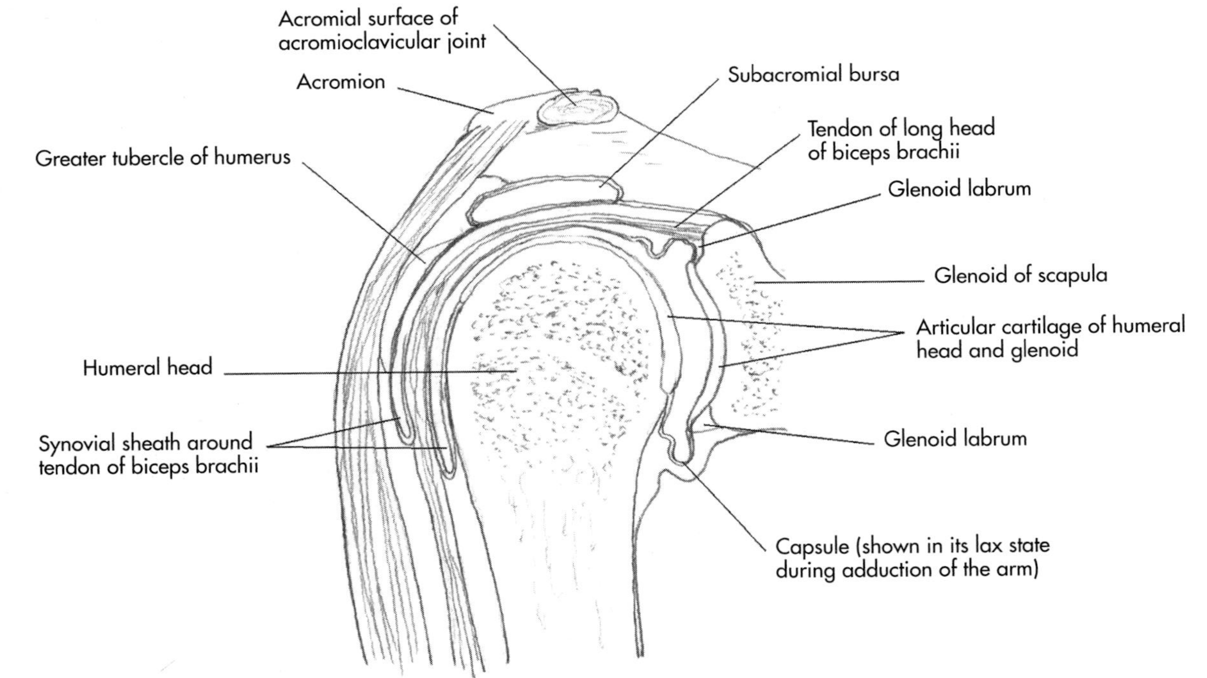

Figure 4.8 Coronal section of the shoulder joint

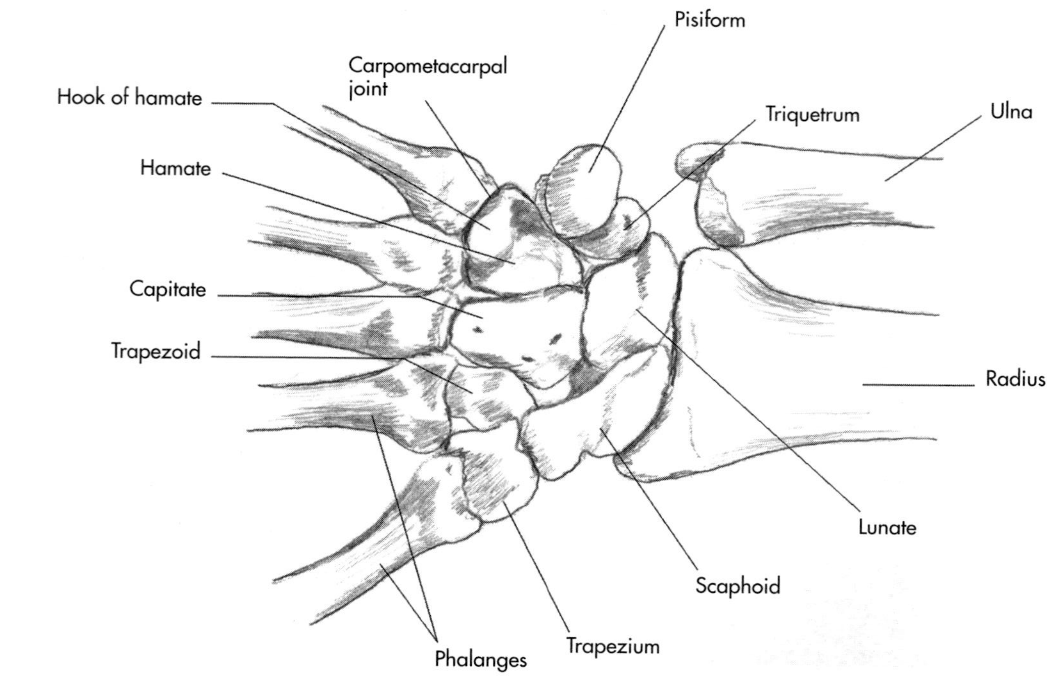

Figure 4.9 Bones of the wrist

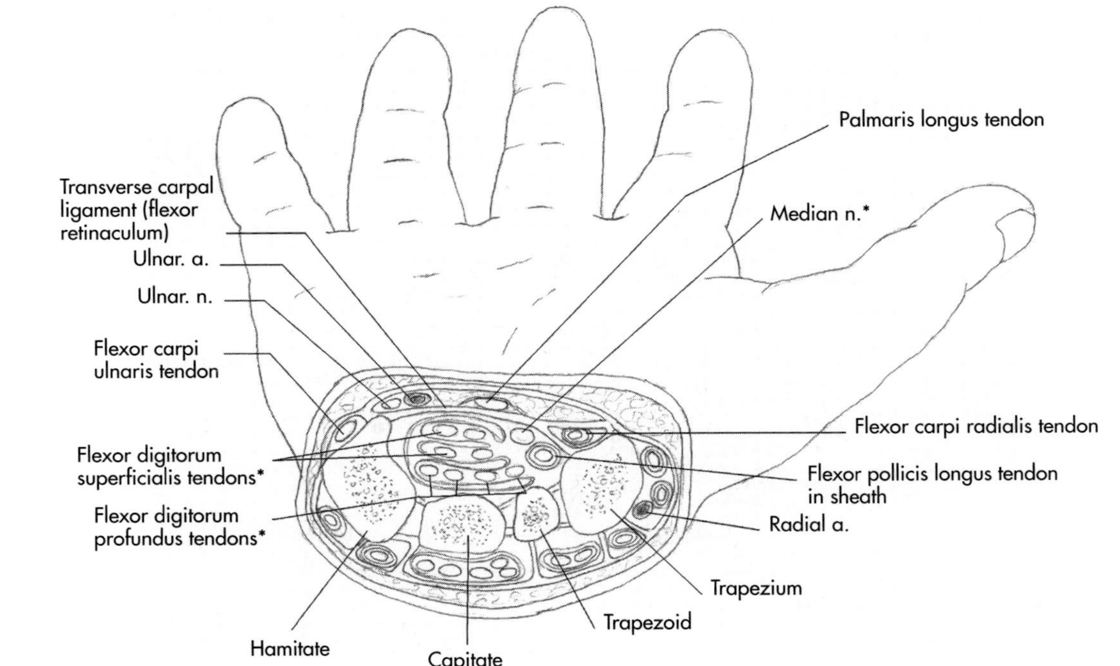

Figure 4.10 Cross-section through the carpal tunnel (contents of the carpal tunnel denoted by an asterisk [*])

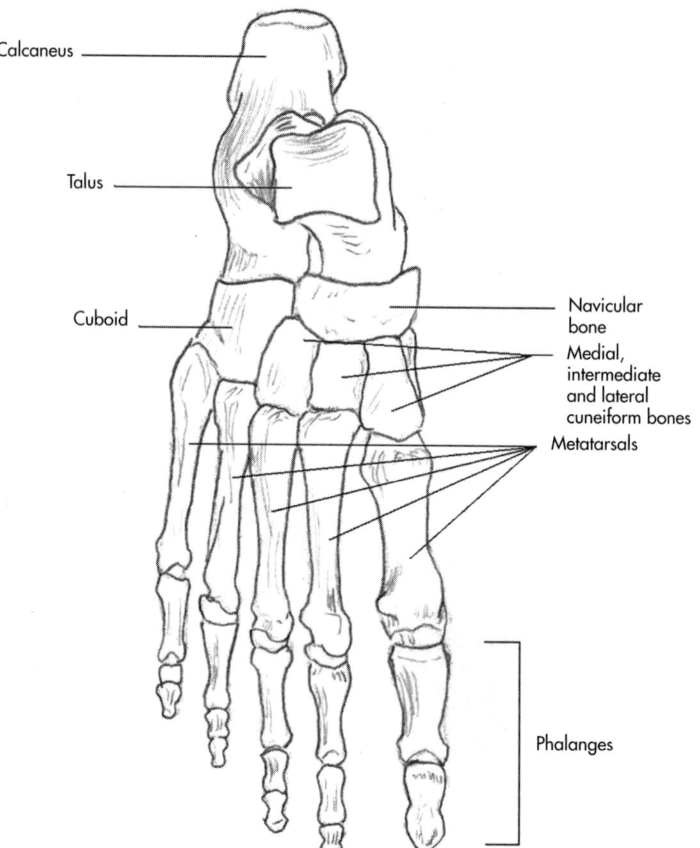

Figure 4.11 Foot bones

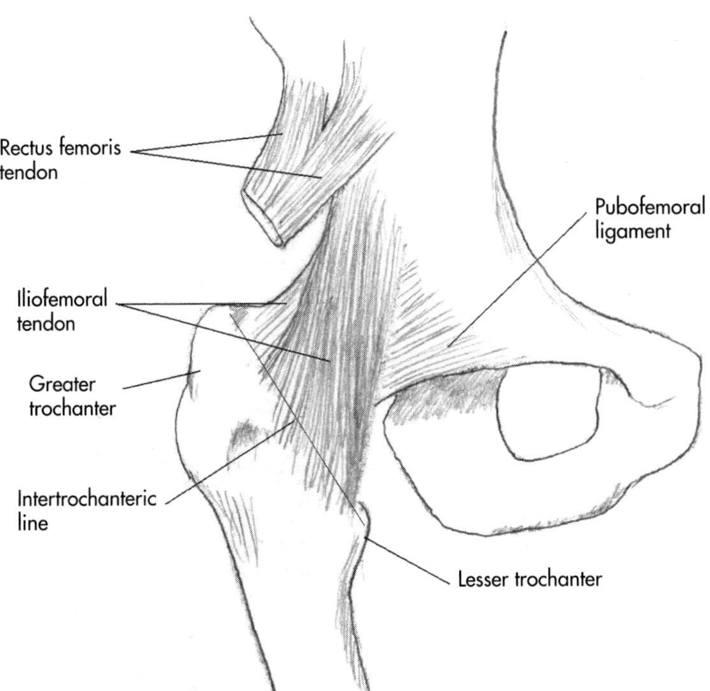

Figure 4.12 Hip joint ligaments

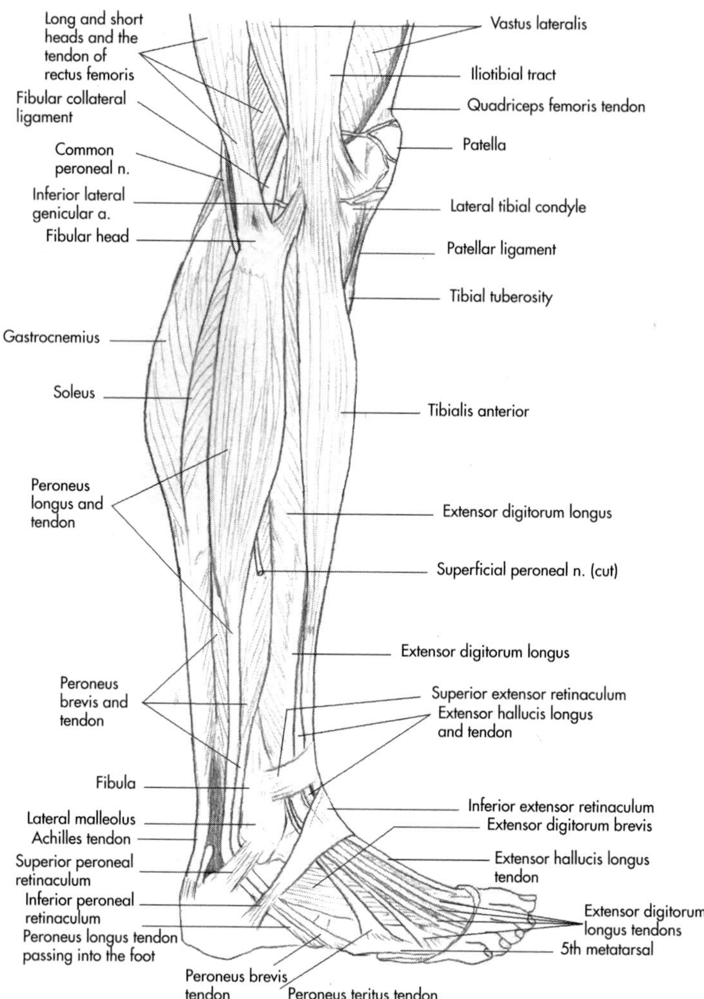
Long and short heads and the tendon of rectus femoris
Fibular collateral ligament
Common peroneal n.
Inferior lateral genicular a.
Fibular head
Gastrocnemius
Soleus
Peroneus longus and tendon
Peroneus brevis and tendon
Fibula
Lateral malleolus
Achilles tendon
Superior peroneal retinaculum
Inferior peroneal retinaculum
Peroneus longus tendon passing into the foot
Peroneus brevis tendon
Peroneus teritus tendon
Vastus lateralis
Iliotibial tract
Quadriceps femoris tendon
Patella
Lateral tibial condyle
Patellar ligament
Tibial tuberosity
Tibialis anterior
Extensor digitorum longus
Superficial peroneal n. (cut)
Extensor digitorum longus
Superior extensor retinaculum
Extensor hallucis longus and tendon
Inferior extensor retinaculum
Extensor digitorum brevis
Extensor hallucis longus tendon
Extensor digitorum longus tendons
5th metatarsal

Figure 4.13 Lateral view of the leg and foot

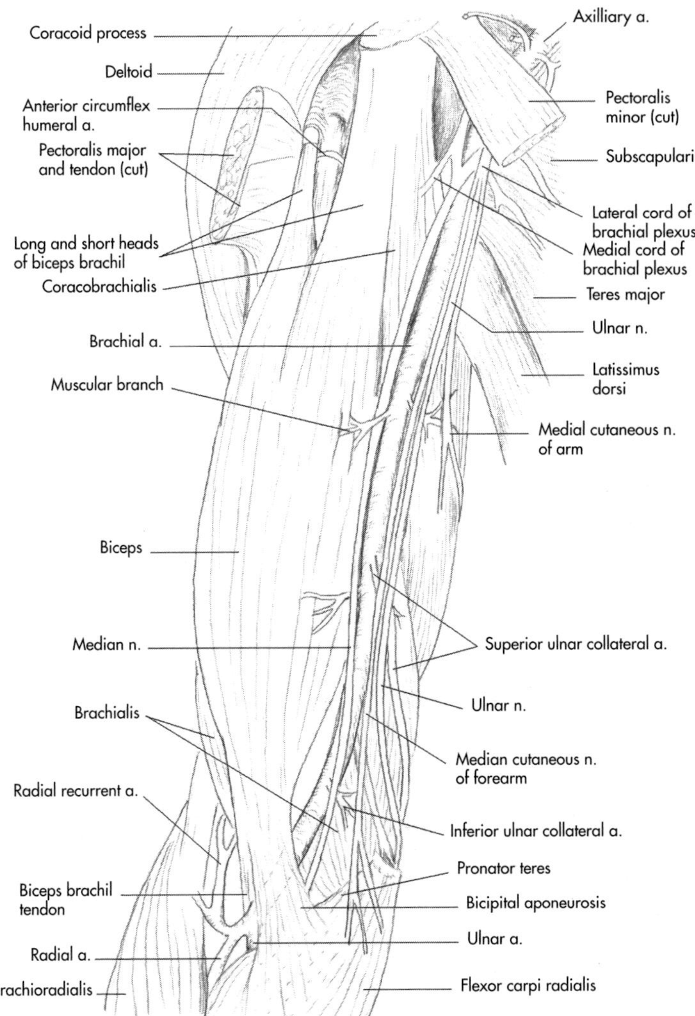

Figure 4.14 Brachial artery and nerves of the upper limb

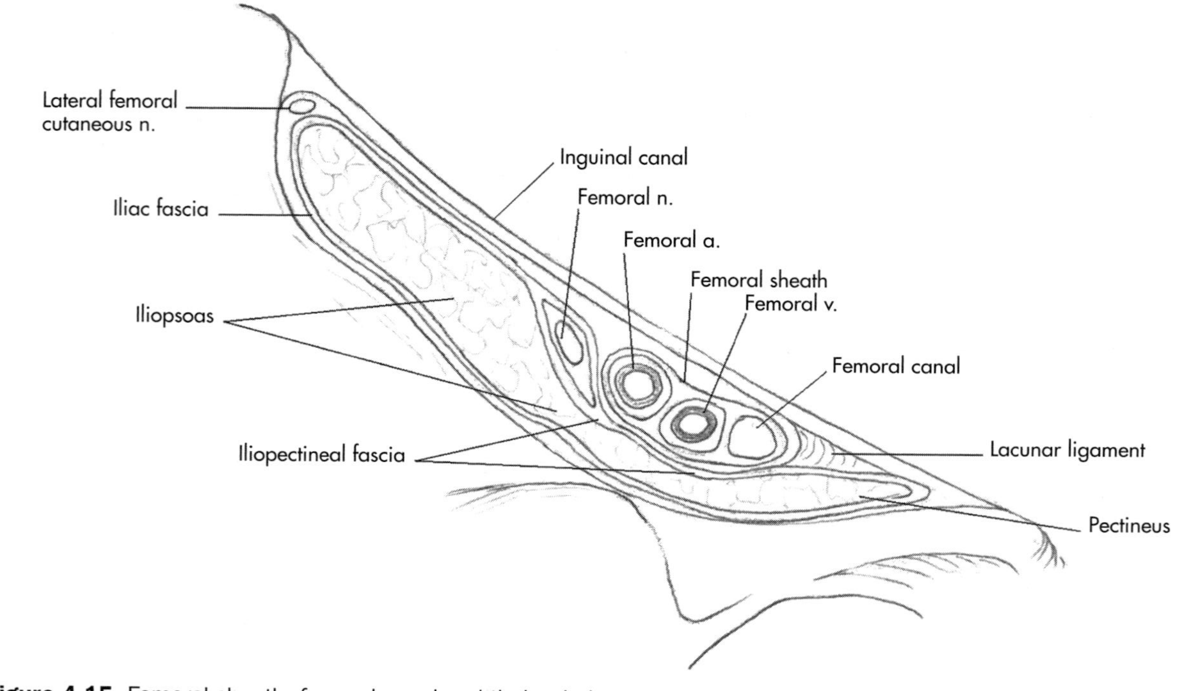

Figure 4.15 Femoral sheath, femoral canal and their relations

CHAPTER 5: CENTRAL NERVOUS SYSTEM

What are the layers of the scalp?

Skin.
Connective tissue.
Aponeurosis.
Loose connective tissue.
Periosteum.
(*Mnemonic:* **SCALP**.)

What is the nerve supply of the scalp?

Greater occipital/**G**reater auricular.
Lesser occipital.
Auriculotemporal.
Supratrochlear.
Supraorbital.
(*Mnemonic:* **GLASS**.)

What bones make up the skull?

Frontal, parietal, occipital, temporal, sphenoid, ethmoid, inferior nasal concha, lacrimal, vomer, nasal, zygomatic, maxilla, palatine, mandible.
Skull bones are joined at sutures and subdivided into the **cranium** (vault [upper] and base of skull [lower]) and the **facial skeleton**.

Which bones make up the base of the skull?

The following:
1. Roof of the orbit (frontal bone).
2. Cribriform plate (ethmoid bone).
3. Sphenoid bone.
4. Squamous and petrous parts of temporal the bone.
5. Occipital bones.

What are the openings in the base of the skull and what structures pass through them?

See Table 5.1.

Table 5.1

Cranial fossa	Opening	Structures passing through
Anterior	Cribriform plate	CN I (olfactory n.)
Middle	Foramen ovale Foramen rotundum Foramen spinosum Foramen lacerum	CN V3 (mandibular division of trigeminal n.) Lesser petrosal n. CN V2 (maxillary division of trigeminal n.) Middle meningeal a. and v. Internal carotid a. Greater petrosal n.
	Optic canal	CN II (optic n.) Ophthalmic a.
	Superior orbital fissure	Frontal, lacrimal and nasociliary nerves, all branches of CN V1 (ophthalmic branch of trigeminal n.) CN III (oculomotor n.), both branches CN IV (trochlear n.) CN VI (abducent n.) Superior ophthalmic v. Sympathetic nn.
Posterior	Foramen magnum Hypoglossal canal Internal acoustic meatus	Medulla oblongata CN XI (spinal accessory n.) Vertebral aa. CN XII (hypoglossal n.) CN VII (facial n.) CN VIII (vestibulocochlear n.) Internal jugular v. (forms from sigmoid sinus)

How are structures passing through the superior orbital fissure remembered?

Sit **N**aked **I**n **A**nticipation **O**f **S**auce.)
Lacrimal nerve.
Frontal nerve.
Trochlear nerve.
Superior branch of oculomotor nerve.
Nasociliary nerve.
Inferior branch of oculomotor nerve.
Abducent nerve.
Ophthalmic veins.
Sympathetic nerves.
(*Mnemonic:* **L**uscious **F**ried **T**omatoes

OSTEOLOGY

What are the sutures of the skull?

Coronal: parietal and parietal bones.
Sagittal: parietal bones.
Lamboid: parietal and occipital bones.
Bregma: sagittal suture and coronal suture.
Lambda: lambda suture and sagittal suture.

What are fontanelles?

At birth ossification is incomplete at both the anterior and posterior fontanelles, the anterior lying at the bregma and the posterior at the lambda artery. They are useful in assessing hydration in a neonate. The other fontanelles are the sphenoidal and the mastoid.

What are the views of the skull?

Norma verticalis.
Norma occipitalis.
Norma frontalis.
Norma lateralis.
Norma basalis.

What bones form the orbit?

Maxillary.
Zygomatic.
Parietal.
Lacrimal.
Ethmoid.
Greater wing of sphenoid.
Orbital plate of frontal bone.

What is contained in the petrous part of the temporal bone?

Middle and inner ear.

What is the nerve supply of the scalp?

Anterior aspect:
- supratrochlear (ophthalmic – frontal)
- supraorbital (ophthalmic – frontal)
- zygomaticotemporal (maxillary).

Posterior aspect:
lesser occipital C2
greater occipital C2.

What is the forebrain, midbrain and hindbrain?

Forebrain:
cerebral hemispheres.
Midbrain:
cerebral peduncles
superior and inferior colliculi.
Hindbrain:
pons
cerebellar hemispheres
medulla.

Why are the ventricles important?

The ventricles are continuous with each other and the central canal. Within the ventricles is the choroid plexus that produces the cerebrospinal fluid (CSF) that circulates in the subarachnoid space.

Where is the CSF reabsorbed?

At the arachnoid granulations lining the venous sinuses.

What bones form the cranial fossa?

Anterior:
orbital plate
cribriform plate
ethmoid bone
lesser wings of the sphenoid bone.
Middle:
lesser wings of the sphenoid bone
squamous part of the temporal bone
greater wing of sphenoid bone
petrous part of the temporal bone.
Posterior:
petrous part of the temporal bone
occipital bone.
(The tentorium cerebella form the roof.)

Where is the pituitary fossa located?

Centrally in the middle cranial fossa in the body of the sphenoid bone.

Which nerves pass through the superior orbital fissure?

Three nerves enter the orbit above the lateral rectus muscle and lie between the roof of the orbit and the orbital muscles. They are branches of the ophthalmic nerve:

Trochlear
Frontal
Lacrimal.

(*Mnemonic:* **T**wo **F**at **L**adies.)

Five structures enter the orbit below and are as follows from lateral to medial from above down:

Superior division of oculomotor nerve
Nasociliary from ophthalmic nerve
Inferior division of oculomotor nerve
Abducent nerve
Ophthalmic veins.

(*Mnemonic:* **S**ip **N**ice **I**nnocent **A**ffordable **V**odkas.)

What are the structures passing through the cavernosus sinus?

Structures are divided into those passing in the lateral wall and into the medial wall:

oculomotor nerve – CN III	Lateral wall
trochlear – CN IV	Lateral wall
ophthalmic – CN V1	Lateral wall
maxillary – CN V2	Lateral wall
abducent – CN VI	Medial wall
internal carotid artery.	Medial wall

Which structures pass through the foramen ovale?

Otic ganglion (lies just inferior).
Lesser superficial petr**O**sal nerve.
Mandibular nerve of trigeminal (**V**3).
Accessory meningeal artery.
Meningeal **L**ymphatics.
Emissary vein.
(*Mnemonic:* **OVALE**.)

Which structures pass through the foramen magnum?

Spinal cord.
Meninges.
Lymphatics.

Accessory nerves (spinal roots).
Sympathetic plexus on vertebral arteries.
Vertebral arteries.
Spinal branches of vertebral arteries.

THE MENINGES

What are the membranes that surround the brain and spinal cord?

There are three membranes that surround the brain and spinal cord. These three layers are the **dura mater**, the **arachnoid mater** and the **pia mater**, and are known as the meninges, which **PAD** the brain (*mnemonic*):

- **P**ia (innermost)
- **A**rachnoid (middle)
- **D**ura (outer): tough and thick, restricts the movement of the brain within the skull, which protects the brain from movements that may cause vascular damage.

Are these layers known by other terms?

Yes. Clinically the dura mater is often called the pachymeninx and the arachnoid and pia mater are called the leptomeninges.

What is the dura mater?

This is a dense, strong fibrous membrane that covers the brain. It has two layers – one adherent to the inner surface of the skull (equivalent to periosteum) called the endosteal layer. The inner layer is the meningeal layer. The meningeal layer is continuous with the dura mater surrounding the spinal cord.

What is the falx cerebri?

This is a fold of dura mater that lies in the midline between the cerebral hemispheres. The superior sagittal sinus runs in its upper margin, the inferior sagittal sinus runs in its lower free border and the straight sinus runs along its attachment with the tentorium cerebelli.

What is the tentorium cerebelli?

This is a fold of dura mater that roofs over the posterior cranial fossa. Its anterior surface is attached to the petrous temporal bone. The superior petrosal sinus runs along this attachment. Laterally it is attached to the occipital bones. In this attachment lie the transverse sinuses (right and left).

What is the nerve supply to the dura mater?

The dura mater is responsive to stretching. The supply is from the trigeminal nerve and the first three cervical nerves. Above the tentorium the dura is innervated by the trigeminal nerve and any pain is referred to the face and forehead. Below the tentorium the supply is from the first three cervical nerves and so any pain is referred to the back of the head and the neck.

Is there a space between the meninges?

Yes. Between the dura and the arachnoid (the middle layer) is the **subdural space**. Between the arachnoid and the pia mater lies the **subarachnoid space**. CSF is present in the subarachnoid space.

Is the subarachnoid space present only around the brain and spinal cord?

No. In addition to these, the arachnoid forms a sheath around the optic nerve. It extends into the orbital cavity and then fuses with the sclera. Therefore, the subarachnoid space extends up to the eyeball.

What are the functions of the meninges?

The meninges, falx and CSF all serve to protect the brain from damage caused by excessive movement.

THE ARTERIAL BLOOD SUPPLY OF THE BRAIN

Does the occipital cortex receive a blood supply from the middle cerebral artery?

Yes.

What is its main blood supply?

Anterior circulation: internal carotid artery (ICA) divides into anterior and middle cerebral arteries. Mainly supplies frontal, temporal, and parietal lobes as well as the deep grey matter.
Posterior circulation: vertebral arteries join to form the basilar artery, which divides into two posterior cerebral arteries. The vertebral artery also gives off the anterior spinal artery of the spinal cord and the posterior inferior cerebellar artery (PICA). The basilar artery gives off the anterior inferior cerebellar artery (AICA) and the superior cerebellar artery (SCA). Branches of the basilar artery supply mainly the pons, cerebellum and thalamus and the posterior cerebral arteries supply the occipital lobes.

What is the circle of Willis?

An arterial anastomosis. The anterior communicating artery between the two anterior cerebral arteries and the two posterior communicating arteries between the internal carotid and posterior cerebral arteries form anastomoses between the anterior and posterior circulations as well as between the left and right systems.

Why is the circle of Willis important?

It has been shown that the blood supply to half the brain is derived from the ipsilateral internal carotid and vertebral arteries. The streams

	from these arteries come together in the posterior communicating artery at a point where the pressure of the two streams is equal. Hence, there is no mixing of blood. However, if there is flow limitation from either artery, the change in pressure allows flow backwards or forwards across that point and compensates for the reduced blood flow. A similar situation also allows flow across the midline to compensate for changes in pressure.
What is its venous drainage?	**Superficial system:** the superior sagittal sinus joins the straight sinus, which forms transverse and sigmoid sinuses that exit the skull as the internal jugular vein (IJV). It drains the cortex and subcortical white matter. **Deep system:** the internal cerebral veins and inferior sagittal sinus drain into the straight sinus.
Where do the venous sinuses lie?	Within the folds of the dura mater.
What are the names of the cranial venous sinuses?	Superior and inferior sagittal sinuses. Great cerebral vein. Straight sinus. Transverse sinus. Superior and inferior petrosal sinuses.
Why is the cavernous sinus significant?	There are communications of the cavernous sinus with facial, ophthalmic veins and the pterygoid plexus, providing a possible pathway for infections on the face to spread to the sinus and on to the superficial middle cerebral vein.

In which intracranial fossa does the cavernous sinus lie?

Middle cranial fossa.

Which structures run above the roof of the cavernous sinus?

Middle cerebral artery.
Optic nerve.

Which structures are medial to the cavernous sinus?

Pituitary fossa and gland within it.
Sphenoid sinus.

What is the main cause of a cavernous sinus thrombosis?

Infection of the facial skin through venous drainage from the face via the orbit.

What are the clinical signs of a cavernous sinus thrombosis?

Ophthalmoplegia: paralysis or weakness of the muscles passing through the sinus that control eye movements .
Chemosis: swelling of the conjunctiva.
Pain.

Which arteries supply blood to the brain?

The arterial supply to the brain comes from the two internal carotid arteries and the two vertebral arteries. The two vertebral arteries join to form the basilar artery. The arteries lie within the subarachnoid space.

What are the areas of the brain supplied by the major branches?

Anterior cerebral artery: remains on the medial surfaces of the frontal and parietal lobes, running upwards and over the corpus callosum. It supplies the orbital surface of the frontal lobe and the medial surface of the cerebral hemisphere.
Middle cerebral artery: passes laterally in the lateral cerebral sulcus. It supplies the lateral surface of the cerebral hemispheres.
Posterior cerebral artery: winds around the cerebral peduncles, reaching the inferior surface of the

occipital lobe. It supplies the lobe and the cortical areas around the calcarine sulcus (visual perception).

What is an extradural haemorrhage?

This is a bleed caused by damage to meningeal arteries or veins. The bleed causes the meningeal dura mater to strip away from the internal surface of the skull. This results in the classic lentiform or biconcave appearance of the extradural haemorrhage on computed tomography (CT). It is most commonly caused by damage to the middle meningeal artery, usually as a result of trauma. The anterior division of the middle meningeal artery is most commonly involved. A skull fracture is present in over 90% of adults with an extradural haemorrhage.

What is a subdural haemorrhage?

This results from the tearing of bridging veins that travel between the cortical surface and the venous sinuses in the subdural space and can result from minor trauma. Elderly people and people with dementia are at greater risk as a result of shrinkage of the brain. This results in a slightly larger gap for the veins to traverse and relatively more brain movement. This is more common than haemorrhage from the middle meningeal artery and is bilateral in approximately 50% of cases.

Through which foramen does the middle meningeal artery enter the skull?

Foramen spinosum, subsequently dividing into anterior and posterior branches.

What clinical finding after a head injury would suggest an extradural haemorrhage?

Anterior branch: hemiplegia.
Posterior branch: deafness.

What region of the skull does the anterior branch run beneath?

The pterion (the weakest part of the skull): the approximation of parietal, frontal temporal and occipital bones.

Why is it important to know the surface markings of the anterior and posterior branches of the middle meningeal artery?

These are the sites where burr holes are made to evacuate the haematoma and reduce the intracranial pressure.

What are the surface markings of the middle meningeal artery?

Anterior division: 3 cm above the midpoint of the zygomatic arch.
Posterior division: where a vertical line from the mastoid process meets a horizontal line from the supraorbital margin.

Can you name some cerebral artery syndromes and their features?

Anterior cerebral artery occlusion. If occlusion is proximal to the anterior communicating artery, there is often adequate preservation of the circulation. If the occlusion is distal to the communicating artery, then the following signs may occur:

- personality change, apathy and inability to identify objects
- contralateral hemiparesis and hemisensory loss mainly affecting the lower limb.

Middle cerebral artery occlusion. The following signs may occur:

- contralateral homonymous hemianopia
- aphasia (if left hemisphere is affected mainly and rarely if the right is affected)
- anosognosia (if right hemisphere is affected mainly and rarely if left is affected)
- contralateral hemiparesis and hemisensory loss, mainly affecting the face and upper limb.

Posterior cerebral artery occlusion.
The following signs may occur:

- contralateral homonymous hemianopia; there may be sparing of the macula to varying degrees
- impairment of memory
- visual agnosia (damage to the left occipital lobe).

Vertebrobasilar artery occlusion.
The clinical signs and symptoms from occlusion in this system are highly complex and eponymous syndromes abound. The symptoms can include the following:

- ipsilateral cerebellar signs
- ipsilateral Horner's syndrome
- ipsilateral pain + temperature loss in the face and contralateral pain + temperature loss in the body
- damage to the vagal and glossopharyngeal nuclei can result in ipsilateral loss of the gag reflex, dysphagia and hoarse voice
- other symptoms include vertigo, nystagmus, coma and hemiparesis.

Of what are the posterior cerebral arteries branches?

The basilar artery.

Which arterial system is involved in a cerebral infarct?

The internal carotid system.

Which arterial system is involved in a brainstem infarct?

The vertebral system.

What is Wallenberg's syndrome?

This syndrome, also known as **lateral medullary syndrome**, can result from occlusion of the PICA. It results in crossed signs and these include ipsilateral ataxia, nystagmus, Horner's syndrome, and involvement of cranial nerves V, VI, VII and VIII and bulbar palsy. There is contralateral pain and temperature loss.

Where do aneurysms tend to occur?

Congenital aneurysms are found most commonly at the junction between two arteries that form the circle of Willis. Aneurysms can be solitary or can occur as part of a syndrome such as polycystic kidney disease.

What are Charcot–Bouchard aneurysms?

These are small microaneurysms approximately 0.8–1.0 mm in diameter. Rupture of these is associated with intracerebral haemorrhage.

THE CEREBELLUM

What is the gross anatomical structure of the cerebellum?

The cerebellum is made up of two hemispheres and a median connecting vermis. It is found in the posterior cranial fossa and forms the roof of the fourth ventricle. It has three main lobes – anterior, middle and flocculonodular. The cerebellum is connected mainly with the same side of the body, so damage will result in ipsilateral signs.

What happens if the vermis is damaged?

This results in signs and symptoms concerned with the midline body structures, i.e. the trunk, neck. These people have difficulty standing or sitting unsupported and they demonstrate truncal ataxia.

What is the function of the cerebellum?

The function of the cerebellum is best thought of as a comparator – it receives input from the cerebral hemispheres, vestibular organs, proprioceptive information from muscles and joints, and possibly also from visual input. It can then influence movement via lower motor neurone activity to achieve the desired outcome. The symptoms associated with cerebellar disease can best be understood if this is remembered.

What are the signs of cerebellar disease?

The mnemonic **VANISH'D** is often used to remember the signs.
Vertigo.
Ataxia: inability to coordinate movements; the ataxic gait is broad-based and the patient staggers and falls to the side of the lesion.
Nystagmus: this is basically ataxia of the eyes. Fast phase towards the lesion.
Intention tremor: the loss of coordinating ability results in a tremor that worsens the nearer the hand approaches the object because this is when the greatest amount of feedback and correlation is required.
Staccato speech: this is essentially ataxia of the muscles of the larynx.
Hypotonia.
Dysdiadochokinesia: inability to perform rapid alternating movements.

What is Holmes' rebound phenomenon?

People with cerebellar lesions are unable to stop strong contractions after the sudden removal of resistance. This is known as Holmes' rebound phenomenon.

What imaging modality is better for visualising the cerebellum?

Although CT and magnetic resonance imaging (MRI) are useful for looking at different things, it is generally accepted that MRI is better for visualising posterior fossa structures.

Can you name some causes of cerebellar syndromes?

Demyelination, e.g. multiple sclerosis.
Stroke/vascular pathology.
Alcoholic degeneration.
Hypothyroidism (reversible).
Paraneoplastic syndromes.
Space-occupying lesions within the posterior fossa.
Friedreich's ataxia.

What is Dandy–Walker syndrome?

Cerebellar hypoplasia and obstruction to the outflow of the fourth ventricle, resulting in infantile hydrocephalus.

What is Arnold–Chiari malformation?

Elongation of the medulla and descent of the cerebellar tonsils into the cervical canal. This condition is associated with spina bifida and patients can develop syringomyelia.

What is the CPA?

CPA stands for cerebellopontine angle. This is a triangular fossa that lies among the cerebellum, lateral pons and the inner third of the petrous temporal bone.

Which nerves are involved with CPA disease?

The cranial nerves V, VI and VII are involved.

What disease processes give rise to this cluster of signs?

Many diseases can cause this pattern. Acoustic neuroma, a schwannoma, is one of the more common. It can be solitary or occur as part of a wider disease process, e.g. type 2 neurofibromatosis.

THE CEREBRUM

What is the parenchyma and stroma?

The parenchyma is the functional part of an organ. The stroma refers to the supporting tissue of the organ.

Describe the gross appearance of the cerebrum.

The cerebrum is made up of two cerebral hemispheres. These are connected to each other via the corpus callosum. The surface of the cerebrum has many folds (gyri) and these are separated by fissures (sulci). The main sulci are the central, parieto-occipital, lateral and calcarine sulci. These sulci are used as borders for the division of the brain into the four different lobes: frontal, temporal, parietal and occipital.

What is the primary motor area?

The primary motor area is part of the frontal lobe and occupies the pre-central gyrus. This area controls movements on the contralateral side of the body.

What is the primary somaesthetic/sensory area?

This is part of the parietal lobe and occupies the postcentral gyrus. The majority of the sensory information received is from the contralateral side of the body.

What is a homunculus?

This is a human figure superimposed on the surface of the brain to represent the sensorimotor regions of the body there. It can be used to determine the area of the brain affected after sensorimotor loss.

What is Broca's area?

This is a part of the inferior frontal lobe on the dominant hemisphere that is involved in the production of speech. Broca's area is close to the primary motor areas of the larynx, mouth, tongue and soft palate, and has connections with these areas. Damage to this area will result in an expressive dysphasia. Patients are able to think the words that they wish to say and can write and are able to understand the written and spoken word, but have difficulty saying the intended word.

What is Wernicke's area?

This is part of the superior temporal gyrus of the temporal lobe in the dominant hemisphere. It receives inputs from the visual and auditory cortex. It is connected to Broca's area via the arcuate fasciculus. Wernicke's area is concerned with the understanding of spoken and written language.

Damage to this area will produce an inability to understand language in either its spoken or written forms. However, as Broca's area is unaffected, the patient will still be able to produce words. Patients are unaware of their meaning and hence use incorrect or made-up words. They are also unaware of any mistakes that they make.

What causes global aphasia?

Damage to both Wernicke's and Broca's areas will result in an inability to understand language and to produce it.

What are the disorders associated with the different lobes of the cerebrum?

See Table 5.2.

What Is Anton's syndrome?

This is cortical blindness. The patient is blind but lacks insight into the severity of the visual loss and commonly denies it. They have normal pupillary responses. It is caused by extensive bilateral damage to the occipital cortex.

What are the names and functions of the 12 cranial nerves?

See Table 5.3.

Table 5.2

Lobe	Dominant hemisphere	Non-dominant hemisphere	Either hemisphere
Frontal	Broca's dysphasia Perserveration Primitive reflexes		Intellectual impairment
Parietal	Limb apraxia	Dressing apraxia Inability to recognise faces	Neglect of opposite limbs Contralateral sensory loss Homonymous field defect
Temporal	Acalculia Alexia Wernicke's dysphasia Agraphia	Failure to recognise faces Confusional states	Homonymous field defect
Occipital			Visual field defects

How can the cranial nerves be remembered?

(*Mnemonic:* Oh Oh Oh To Touch And Feel Virgin Girls' Vaginas And Hymens.) (In that order, see Table 5.3.)

How is the cranial nerve supply remembered?

(*Mnemonic:* Some Say Marry Money, But My Brother Says Big Brains Matter More.) (In that order, see Table 5.3.)

Table 5.3 Cranial nerves

No.	Nerve	Function	Course and relations	Branches	Type
I	Olfactory	Smell	The olfactory receptor cells in the upper nasal cavity give rise to the olfactory nerve fibres that pass through the cribriform plate of the ethmoid bone to enter the olfactory bulb	–	Sensory
II	Optic	Vision	Optic canal	–	Sensory
III	Oculomotor	Raises upper eyelid Pupil constriction Accommodation Supplies all eye muscles EXCEPT lateral rectus and superior oblique	Nucleus: in the anterior part of the grey matter around the cerebral aqueduct at the level of the superior corpus quadrigeminum. From the anterior surface of midbrain passing forwards with posterior cerebral a. above, superior cerebellar a. below and posterior communicating a. medial. It continues forwards into the middle cranial fossa and pierces the dura of the roof of the cavernous sinus lateral to the posterior clinoid between free and attached borders of the tentorium cerebelli. In the cavernous sinus the nerve lies as the highest structure in the lateral wall, and is then crossed laterally from below upwards by the trochlear n.	It divides into two branches. These pass through the superior orbital fissure into the orbit between the two heads of the lateral rectus m., embracing the nasociliary n. The upper division distributes to levator palpabrae and superior rectus. The lower division distributes to medial rectus, inferior rectus and inferior oblique and gives a motor root to the ciliary ganglion	Motor

Table 5.3 Continued

No.	Nerve	Function	Course and relations	Branches	Type
IV	Trochlear	Assists in turning eye down and medially	Emerges from the posterior surface of the midbrain and immediately decussates with the nerve from the opposite side. It passes through the middle cranial fossa and the cavernous sinus. It then passes into the orbital cavity via the superior orbital fissure to supply the superior oblique m.	–	Motor
V	Trigeminal	**Ophthalmic:** Sensory to skin of forehead, cornea, eyelids and mucous membranes of nasal cavity **Maxillary:** Sensory to upper teeth, skin over maxillary area **Mandibular:** Sensory to lower teeth, side of head and temporomandibular joint. Motor to muscles of mastication	Leaves the anterior pons as a small motor root and a large sensory root. It courses forwards to enter the middle cranial fossa where it rests on the upper surface of the apex of the petrous temporal bone. Here the trigeminal ganglion of the sensory nerve is formed and this is found in Meckel's cave – a sac of dura mater	**Ophthalmic:** Frontal, dividing into supratrochlear and supraorbital nn. Lacrimal Nasociliary Dural Communicating to third, fourth and sixth sympathetics **Maxillary:** Meningeal Ganglionic to sphenopalatine ganglion Zygomatic Dental (posterior, middle, anterior)	

Table 5.3 Cranial nerves (continued)

No.	Nerve	Function	Course and relations	Branches	Type
(V)	(Trigeminal)			Palpebral Labial Nasal **Mandibular:** Nervus sponiosus (trunk) Medial pterygoid (trunk) Lateral pterygoid (anterior division) Temporal (anterior and posterior divisions) Buccal (anterior division) Masseteric (anterior division) Lingual (posterior division) Inferior dental (posterior division) Auriculotemporal (posterior division) The ophthalmic division enters the orbital cavity via the superior orbital fissure. The maxillary nerve exits the skull via the foramen rotundum and the mandibular division leaves via foramen ovale	
VI	Abducent	Moves eye laterally	The nerve passes anteriorly from the pons in the groove between the pons and the medulla and through to the cavernous sinus. It then enters the orbital cavity via the superior orbital fissure and supplies the lateral	–	Motor

Table 5.3 Continued

No.	Nerve	Function	Course and relations	Branches	Type
VII	Facial	**Motor:** Muscles of face and scalp, stapedius, posterior belly of digastric and stylohyoid **Sensory:** Taste from anterior two-thirds of tongue via chorda tympani n. **Secretory:** Submandibular and sublingual glands, lacrimal glands and glands of nose and palate	The nerve has both sensory and motor roots. The motor fibres initially travel posteriorly around the abducent nucleus before travelling anteriorly to emerge with the sensory root from the brainstem between the pons and the medulla. The nerve passes laterally in the posterior fossa with CN VIII and enters the internal acoustic meatus. It then enters the facial canal and travels laterally through the inner ear. After forming the geniculate ganglion the nerve turns backwards sharply. The nerve exits the middle ear via the stylomastoid foramen and passes between the deep and superficial portions of the parotid gland. On reaching the parotid gland the nerve splits into temporofacial and cervicofacial branches that pierce the parotid gland and stimulate the muscles of facial expression	**In temporal bone:** Great superficial petrosal Root to lesser superficial petrosal n. – to otic ganglion External superficial petrosal – to middle meningeal a. Nerve to stapedius Chorda tympani Communicating to vagus Nervus intermedius – greater petrosal to pterygopalatine ganglion **In the neck:** Posterior auricular Posterior belly of digastric Stylohyoid **On the face:** **T**emporal Upper **z**ygomatic Lower **z**ygomatic **B**uccal **M**andibular **C**ervical (*Mnemonic:* **T**wo **Z**ulus **B**uried **M**y **C**at)	Both

Table 5.3 Cranial nerves (continued)

No.	Nerve	Function	Course and relations	Branches	Type
VIII	Vestibulocochlear	**Vestibular:** position and head movements **Cochlear:** hearing	Leave the anterior surface of the brain between the pons and medulla and run laterally within the posterior fossa to enter the internal acoustic meatus	–	Sensory
IX	Glossopharyngeal	**Motor:** Stylopharyngeus – assists in swallowing **Sensory:** Taste – posterior third of tongue and pharynx Carotid sinus (baroreceptors) Carotid body (chemoreceptors) **Secretory:** Parotid gland	Leaves anterolateral surface of medulla and passes laterally through the posterior fossa before exiting via the jugular foramen. It then travels through the neck accompanied by the internal jugular vein and internal carotid artery. At the posterior border of stylopharyngeus it supplies its motor branch. It then passes forwards between the middle and superior constrictors to give off its sensory branches to the pharynx and tongue	Tympanic n. Pharyngeal n. Nerve to stylopharyngeus Lingual Tonsillar	Both

Table 5.3 Continued

No.	Nerve	Function	Course and relations	Branches	Type
X	Vagus	**Sensory:** Inferior pharynx, larynx and abdominal and thoracic viscera **Motor:** Muscles of the soft palate – pharynx, larynx muscles, palatoglossus	The course of the vagus is long and different on the left and right sides. It leaves the anterolateral surface of the medulla and travels through the posterior cranial fossa before leaving via the jugular foramen. Just superior to the jugular foramen is the superior sensory ganglion and just inferior to the jugular foramen is the inferior sensory ganglion. It travels down through the neck within the carotid sheath and then the left and right nerves follow different paths The **right vagus** enters the thorax and passes posterior to the hilum of the right lung. It then passes posteriorly on to the posterior surface of the oesophagus before entering the abdomen via the oesophageal opening in the diaphragm The **left vagus** enters the thorax and crosses the aortic arch before descending posterior to the left lung hilum. It descends along the anterior surface of the oesophagus and enters the abdomen via the oesophageal opening in the diaphragm	Meningeal n. Auricular n. Pharyngeal n. Superior laryngeal (subdivides into internal and external) Recurrrent laryngeal Cardiac Anterior and posterior pulmonary Oesophageal Gastric Pancreatic Intestinal Splenic Hepatic	Both

Table 5.3 Cranial nerves (continued)

No.	Nerve	Function	Course and relations	Branches	Type
XI	Accessory	Sternocleidomastoid and trapezius	The fibres emerge from the first five cervical roots. These nerve fibres then ascend up through the foramen magnum where they join cranial nerve X. The fibres then pass laterally through the jugular foramen and travel along the internal carotid artery. It enters the deep surface of sternocleidomastoid and travels to the posterior triangle to supply trapezius The cranial roots quickly combine with the vagus n. The cranial part of CN XI can be thought of contributing entirely to the vagus n.	–	Motor
XII	Hypoglossal	Muscles of the tongue (except palatoglossus)	Fibres emerge from the anterior surface of the medulla and travel through the posterior fossa to exit the cranial cavity via the hypoglossal canal. It then descends along with the internal carotid a. before looping back to pass the mandible medially and inferiorly. It then enters the tongue	**Meningeal:** Communicating to vagus via sympathetic Descending br. with descendens cervicalis forms ansa hypoglossi, which innervates infrahyoid mm. Nerve to thyrohyoid **Lingual:** Geniohyoid n. Genioglossus n. Styloglossus n. Hyoglossus n. Intrinsic mm.	Motor

CHAPTER 6: SENSORY ORGANS

THE ORBIT

What is the orbit?	A bony cavity that contains the eye and its associated structures.
What are the relations of the bony orbit?	**Superior:** frontal bone. **Lateral:** frontal, zygomatic and greater wing of sphenoid bones. **Medial:** frontal, maxillary ethmoid and lacrimal bones. **Inferior:** maxillary and zygomatic bones. **Roof:** frontal bone and lesser wing of sphenoid. **Floor:** zgomatic and maxillary bones.
Where do the optic canal and superior orbital fissure lie?	**Optic canal:** within the lesser wing of the sphenoid, medial to the fissure. **Superior orbital fissure:** between the lesser and greater wings of the sphenoid.
What is a blowout fracture?	An orbital floor fracture after which there in an increased volume of the orbit, resulting in exophthalmos (protrusion of the eye). The inferior rectus muscle or orbital tissue can becomes entrapped within the fracture site, causing tethering and prohibiting the upward movement of the globe, resulting in diplopia. Other complications include emphysema, orbital haemorrhage and retinal damage.
How are the eyelids retracted?	The levator superioris can raise the upper lid independently. Both the upper lids and the lower lids are closed by the orbicularis oculi muscle.

What structures are found in the eyelid?	Skin. Superficial fascia. Orbicularis oculi. Levator superioris. Ciliary glands (sweat glands). Sebaceous glands with eyelashes. Tarsal glands. Conjunctiva.
What are the tarsi?	Two thin plates (upper and lower) of fibrous tissue supporting the eyelids. They are attached to the medial and lateral palpebral ligaments.
What is the conjunctiva?	A mucous membrane lining the eyelids. This layer is continuous with the corneal epithelium of the eye. When swollen, the condition is called chemosis and, when infected, conjunctivitis. Conjunctivitis can be unilateral or bilateral.
What is the lacrimal apparatus?	It consists of the lacrimal gland located in the upper outer aspect of the orbit. The gland secretes tears that drain through the lacrimal canaliculi and sac at the medial aspect of the eye into the nasolacrimal duct, which enters the nose at the inferior meatus.
Where is the lacrimal gland?	In the upper lateral wall of the orbit in the lacrimal fossa.
What is the function of the lacrimal gland?	It is a serous gland that produces tears.
Where do tears drain to?	The nasolacrimal duct at the medial canthus and then into the inferior meatus of the nose.
What are the muscles of eyeball movement and what nerves supply them?	Superior oblique – trochlear nerve. Inferior oblique – oculomotor nerve. Superior rectus – oculomotor nerve. Medial rectus – oculomotor nerve.

Inferior rectus – oculomotor nerve.
Lateral rectus – abducent nerve.

What does $LR_6(SO_4)_3$ mean?

This is a formula for remembering which extraocular muscles are supplied by which nerve. The lateral rectus is supplied by CN VI, the superior oblique by CN IV and all the muscles are supplied by CN III.

What do the ocular muscles attach to?

The tendinous ring (except inferior oblique).

What suspends the eye in the orbit?

Lateral check ligament.
Medial check ligament.
Suspensory ligament of Lockwood.

What enters the orbit?

Superior orbital fissure:

lacrimal – ophthalmic nerve (CN V1)
frontal – ophthalmic nerve (CN V1)
trochlear nerve (CN IV).

Superior orbital fissure within the tendinous ring:

optic nerve (CN II)
ophthalmic artery
nasociliary – ophthalmic nerve (CN V1)
superior and inferior branches of oculomotor nerve (CN III)
abducent nerve (CN VI).

Inferior orbital fissure:

infraorbital – maxillary (CN V2)
zygomatic – maxillary (CN V2).

What is directly related to the superior orbital fissure?

The cavernous sinus.

Why does increased cranial pressure cause papilloedema?

The optic nerve is covered by all layers of the meninges and these are continuous with the intracranial meninges. Any rise in intracranial pressure is transmitted to the subarachnoid space surrounding the optic nerve impeding venous return, leading to swelling the optic disc (papilloedema).

How do you measure visual acuity?

A Snellen chart is read at 6 m (20 feet). The result is expressed as two figures, e.g. 20/20. The first figure represents the distance from the chart and the second the smallest letters read by the patient. The higher the second number, the worse the visual acuity.

Where is the ciliary ganglion located?

A few millimetres lateral to the optic nerve within the orbital fat. It is known as a 'ganglion' as a result of the parasympathetic synapse.

What nerves supply the ganglion?

Oculomotor nerve: preganglionic parasympathetic nerves.
Superior cervical ganglion: postganglionic sympathetic nerves.
Nasociliary nerve (ophthalmic – CN V1): sensory nerves.

What connects the ciliary ganglion to the eye?

The short ciliary nerve.
Note that the nasociliary nerve also supplies separate sympathetic and sensory nerves to the eye via the long ciliary nerve.

What does each nerve from the ciliary ganglion supply?

Parasympathetic:
- sphincter pupillae muscle (constricts pupil)
- ciliary muscle (accommodation).

Sympathetic:
- vessels of eyeball
- sphincter pupillae muscle (dilates pupil).

Sensory:
- eyeball
- cornea.

What signs are seen in complete CN III palsy?

Unilateral complete ptosis.
Eye faces down and out.
A fixed and dilated pupil.

What is the difference between a surgical and a medical CN III palsy?

The parasympathetic supply to the pupil runs on the superior surface of CN III.
Medical CN III palsy: damage to the third nerve, e.g. by infarction, will spare these fibres and hence the pupil will behave normally.
Surgical CN III palsy: extrinsic compression, e.g. by a posterior communicating artery aneurysm, will cause damage to CN III and the parasympathetic nerves that are on its surface. This will result in a dilated pupil and pain.

In which direction of gaze is diplopia maximal in CN VI palsy?

The eye cannot be abducted beyond the midline in CN VI palsy. Therefore, diplopia is maximal on looking towards the side of the lesion.

What sign will be seen in complete CN VI palsy?

The affected eye will be completely adducted because there will be unopposed action of the adductors.

Why is the nerve prone to damage?

It has the longest intradural course within the cranial cavity of all the cranial nerves. It also lies in close apposition to the petrous temporal bone. In raised intracranial pressure, the nerve is compressed against the tip of the petrous temporal bone and this causes a false localising sign.

What is internuclear ophthalmoplegia?

Cranial nerves III and VI are linked via the medial longitudinal fasciculus (MLF). This allows our eyes to move in the horizontal plane in harmony with each other. If the MLF is damaged, when we look left or right, the ipsilateral lateral rectus muscle will contract and abduct the eye but the contralateral CN III will not work, so the opposite eye does not move.

Note that the eyes can still move in all directions if tested individually but they do not do so in coordination with each other.

Why is the central artery of the retina important?

This is a small artery branch of the ophthalmic artery (internal carotid artery), which continues forwards with the optic nerve. It is a terminal artery of the retina. If occluded it can lead to total or partial blindness.

What are the layers of the back of the eye?

Retina (inner).
Choroid (middle), continuous with ciliary body and iris.
Sclera (outer), continuous with the cornea.

What are the chambers of the eye?

Anterior: lies between the cornea and iris; contains aqueous fluid.
Posterior: lies between the iris and the lens; contains aqueous fluid.
Vitreous: lies between the lens and optic nerve, encompassing the rest of the eye. It contains the gelatinous, transparent vitreous body.

What are the layers of the retina?

Ganglion cell layer.
Bipolar cell layer.
Layers of rods and cones.

What are the blind spot, macula lutea and fovea centralis?

Blind spot: the penetration of the optic disc gives a region of the retina that lacks rods and cones.
Macula lutea: lying at the optical axis, rods and cones are numerous in this area.
Fovea centralis: the focus point at the centre of the macula; only cone (colour-sensing) cells are found.

What is glaucoma?

A rise in intraocular pressure. Aqueous humour is formed in the posterior chamber by capillaries of the ciliary body. It is absorbed at the angle between the cornea and iris into the canal of Schlemm in the anterior chamber. Obstruction causes glaucoma. It can be acute or chronic. Symptoms include pain and decreased acuity.

How is the light reflex mediated?

Light shone into the eye will cause constriction of the pupils. The pupil into which the light is shone is the direct reflex and the opposite pupil is the consensual reflex. The pathway is as follows:

Afferent pathway: an image on the retina causes an action potential that travels via the optic nerve to the lateral geniculate bodies. Some of the fibres from the optic nerve decussate at the optic chiasma so that the lateral geniculate bodies receive a bilateral input. The impulse then travels to the pretectal nucleus.

Efferent pathway: the impulse then propagates to each Edinger–Westphal nucleus. From here, via CN III and the ciliary ganglion, the impulse is passed to each pupil and constriction occurs.

How does the accommodation reflex differ?

The accommodation reflex involves change in both the eye position and the pupil. The pathway is similar but not identical to the light reflex. Impulses travel via the optic nerve to the visual cortex. Here the impulses are projected to the frontal eye field. From there, the impulses travel to the oculomotor nerve nuclei via the internal capsule and hence to the medial recti. Some of the fibres also travel to the Edinger–Westphal nucleus bilaterally and then to each pupil via the ciliary ganglion. Hence, the accommodation reflex involves both eye movement and pupil changes.

How is the corneal reflex mediated?

Lightly touching the cornea or conjunctiva will cause blinking. Afferent impulses travel via the ophthalmic division of the trigeminal nerve (V1). Internuncial neurones then connect with the motor nucleus of the facial nerve bilaterally via the MLF. The facial nerve supplies nerves to the orbicularis oculi muscles of the eye, which mediate closure.

What governs the size of the pupils?

Pupil size is governed by the balance of flow to the pupils from its sympathetic and parasympathetic innervation.
Parasympathetic innervation comes via the ciliary nerves and stimulates the sphincter muscle of the pupil, causing the pupils to constrict.
Sympathetic innervation comes via the nasociliary nerves, which arise from the superior cervical ganglion, and cause dilatation of the pupil.

Can you describe some clinical abnormalities of the pupils?

Argyll Robertson pupil
A small irregular pupil that is fixed to light but responds normally to accommodation. Remember the phrase **A**ccommodation **R**eflex **P**resent (**ARP**). Occurs in neurosyphilis and diabetes. (*Mnemonic:* think of a prostitute with syphilis – the prostitute's pupil accommodates but does not react.)
Holmes–Adie pupil
This is also known as a myotonic pupil, and is a dilated pupil that has a slow or no reaction to either light or

accommodation. It is caused by denervation in the ciliary ganglion.

Afferent pupillary defect

A complete transection of the optic nerve on the left will cause:

- loss of direct light response on the left, and
- loss of consensual response on the right.

Relative afferent pupillary defect

Incomplete damage to the afferent pathway can be tested using the swinging light test. If we assume the damage is on the left, then:

- the direct and consensual reflex is present on shining the light into the left eye;
- the consensual reflex is normal on shining the light into the right eye;
- when the light is swung back to the left eye its pupil dilates relative to its previous state.

THE NOSE

What is the function of the nose?

To warm, moisten and filter air.
To smell.

What makes up the external nose?

Nasal bones.
Lateral nasal cartilages.
Greater alar cartilages.
Soft tissue.
Frontal process of maxilla.

What are the boundaries of the nasal cavity?

Floor:

- palatine process of maxilla
- horizontal process of palatine bone.

Roof:

- nasal bone
- frontal bone
- ethmoid bone
- sphenoid bone.

Lateral:
maxillary bone
palatine bone
sphenoid bone
lacrimal bone
ethmoid bone
upper middle and lower conchae.

What are the openings below the concha?

Inferior: nasolacrimal duct.
Middle: hiatus semilunaris (frontonasal duct, anterior ethmoidal sinuses, maxillary sinuses).
Superior: posterior ethmoidal sinuses.
Roof: sphenoethmoidal recess (sphenoidal sinuses).

What makes up the nasal septum?

Septal cartilage (anterior).
Perpendicular plate of the ethmoid bone (posterior).
Vomer (thin sheet of bone).
Nasal crest of the maxilla and palatine bone.

What is the blood supply to the nasal septum?

Anterior ethmoid artery (from ophthalmic artery).
Septal branches of superior labial artery (from facial artery).
Sphenopalatine and ascending branch of the greater palatine artery (from the maxillary artery).

What is the type of epithelium?

Ciliated columnar respiratory, with many mucus-secreting goblet cells.

Where is the olfactory epithelium?

Roof and superior septum in the sphenoethmoidal recess and under the superior concha.

How can the olfactory epithelium be distinguished from the rest of the nasal mucosa?

It has a yellowish colour.

What is the blood supply?	Sphenopalatine (maxillary, external carotid). Anterior and posterior ethmoidal (ophthalmic, internal carotid). Greater palatine (maxillary, external carotid). Superior labial (facial, external carotid). Angular (facial, external carotid).
What is Kiesselbach's plexus (Little's area)?	Little's area represents a region in the anteroinferior third of the nasal septum where all three of the chief blood supplies to the internal nose converge. It is a common site for epistaxis (nose bleed).
What is the nerve supply?	Branches of the ophthalmic and maxillary nerves (CN V1 and V2).

EAR

What is the function of the ear and vestibular apparatus?	Hearing, position and movement of the head.
What are the organs responsible for this function?	Cochlea, semicircular canals and vestibule, all supplied by the vestibulocochlear nerve (CN VIII).
What is the auricle (pinna)?	Consists of the helix, antihelix, lobule, tragus and antitragus. It contains the external acoustic meatus.
What is the sensory supply to the auricle?	Auriculotemporal nerve (mandibular CN V3). Great auricular nerve (C2 – cervical plexus). Auricular branch of the vagus nerve.
What is the function of the pinna?	Amplification and localisation of sound.

What is the external acoustic meatus?	Extending from the auricle, it measures 2.5 cm to the tympanic membrane (eardrum). The outer third consists of cartilage.
What is the middle ear cavity?	A cavity lined by a mucous membrane in the temporal bone.
What are the relations of the middle ear?	**Lateral wall:** tympanic membrane external auditory meatus. **Anterior wall:** carotid canal Eustachian tube. **Medial wall:** inner ear facial nerve. **Posterior wall:** mastoid air cells facial nerve. **Roof:** tegumen tympani and middle cranial fossa. **Floor:** jugular bulb.
What are the contents of the middle ear?	Ossicles. Facial nerve. Tensor tympani muscle (supplied by mandibular nerve). Stapedius muscle (supplied by facial nerve). Chorda tympani (branch of the facial nerve).
What are the names given to the three ossicles?	Malleus. Incus. Stapes.
Which part of the ossicles connects to the tympanic membrane?	The handle of the malleus.
How are the ossicles connected together?	By synovial joints.

What structure does the footplate of the stapes connect to?	The oval window (fenestra vestibuli) of the cochlea. The other window of the cochlea is the fenestra cochleae and is covered by a secondary tympanic membrane.
What are the nerves given off by the facial nerve in the middle ear?	**Greater petrosal nerve:** supplies parasympathetic fibres and joins the deep petrosal nerve to become the nerve of the pterygoid canal, entering into the pterygopalatine ganglion. **Stapedius:** to stapedius muscle of the middle ear. **Chorda tympani:** taste to the anterior two-thirds of the tongue via the lingual nerve.
What is the function of the muscles in the middle ear?	Reduce the movement of the ossicles to avoid over-vibration during low-pitch and loud noises.
What is the main nerve supply to the middle ear?	Glossopharyngeal nerve (this is why there is often referred pain to the ears in tonsillitis).
Where does the auditory (Eustachian) tube open?	It opens high in the nasopharynx by perforating the pharyngobasilar fascia above the superior constrictor muscle. It arrives from the middle ear, acting as a pressure equaliser between the two cavities on yawning and swallowing. The muscle responsible is tensor veli palatini.
What happens if the Eustachian tube is not able to open (e.g. with enlarged adenoids or during a middle ear infection)?	The pressure difference means that the tympanic membrane cannot move in response to sound, so there is reduced hearing on the affected side; it is often associated with pain. If the pressure difference is large this can cause perforation of the eardrum.

How many layers does the tympanic membrane have?

Three:
inner, columnar
middle, fibrous
outer, stratified squamous.

In what structure does the internal ear lie?

The petrous part of the temporal bone. It forms a bony labyrinth. Within this labyrinth lies a membranous labyrinth following the course of the bony cavity. Between the membrane and the bone is perilymph. The membranous labyrinth is filled with **endolymph**.

What structures comprise the inner ear and what are their functions?

Cochlear: hearing accomplished by the spiral organ of Corti.
Semicircular canals: rotational acceleration (balance while head is in motion).
Utricle and saccule of the vestibule: linear acceleration and gravity (balance while the head is still).

What are the otolith organs?

The **utricle** and **saccule**. They are structures of the vestibular labyrinth that are sensitive to linear acceleration and gravity. The utricle is sensitive to a change in horizontal movement, and the saccule is sensitive to vertical acceleration. Otoliths are small particles of calcium carbonate in the viscous fluid of the saccule and utricle. They stimulate the hair cells and consequently the nerve on movement.

What are Rinne's and Weber's tests?

Rinne's test
Looking for sensorineural deafness: mastoid vibration is better.
Looking for failure of conduction: mastoid vibration is better.

Weber's test
Looking for sensorineural deafness: the vibrations localise to the side of the normal cochlea.
Looking for conductive deafness: the vibrations localise to the affected ear.

What are caloric tests?

These are tests that are used to assess vestibular function. They involve putting water of various temperatures into the external auditory meatus. This then causes convection currents to form in the endolymph of the semicircular canals, which are detected by the vestibular nerve.
The normal caloric test is as follows:

- ice cold water in the left ear causes nystagmus with the fast phase to the RIGHT;
- warm water in the left ear causes nystagmus with the fast phase to the LEFT;
- and vice versa.

Changes in this response are caused by damage to the labyrinth (ipsilateral side), CN VIII or brainstem.

What is nystagmus?

It is a series of involuntary oscillations of one or both eyes. The oscillations are rhythmic and can be horizontal, vertical or rotatory in direction.

What symptoms are associated with cochlear nerve damage?

Tinnitus and sensorineural deafness.

ORAL CAVITY

What is the tongue?

A mobile muscular organ covered by epithelium.

How is it divided?	The anterior two-thirds lie in the oral cavity and the posterior third lies in the oropharynx.
What is the frenulum?	A fold on the ventral surface of the tongue covered with smooth epithelium. It is seen if the tongue is raised. The submandibular and sublingual ducts and the deep lingual veins arise lateral to this.
What are the structures on the dorsal surface of the tongue?	**Filiform and fungiform papillae:** taste buds. **Sulcus terminalis:** a V-shaped groove separating the anterior two-thirds from the posterior third. **Foramen caecum:** a pit at the tip of the aforementioned 'V'. Indicates the site of the proximal end of the thyroglossal duct. **Circumvallate papillae:** just anterior to the sulcus terminalis; carry copious taste buds. **Lingual tonsil:** the epithelium behind the sulcus terminalis is composed of this lymphoid tissue, otherwise known as the lymphoid tonsil.
Which nerve supplies taste to the anterior two-thirds of the tongue?	Chorda tympani (from the facial nerve in the middle ear) which accompanies the lingual nerve.
Which nerve supplies sensation to the anterior two-thirds of the tongue?	Lingual nerve (mandibular CN V2).
Which nerve supplies sensation and taste to the posterior third of the tongue?	Glossopharyngeal nerve (CN IX).
What nerve supplies the muscles of the tongue?	Hypoglossal nerve (CN XII) supplies the intrinsic and extrinsic muscles of the tongue.

Where are the extrinsic muscles attached?	Bony attachments, including the palate, styloid process, hyoid bone and mandible.
What is the blood supply to the tongue?	Lingual artery, a branch of the external carotid artery. It runs deep to the hyoglossus to reach the tip of the tongue.
What is important about the lymphatic drainage of the tongue?	There is crossover so that lymph drains to nodes bilaterally. This is significant in the spread of cancer in this region.
In which direction does the tongue protrude if the nerve is damaged?	The tongue will protrude TOWARDS the side of the lesion as a result of muscle paralysis. The intact muscles push the tongue to the side of weakness.
What are the parts of a tooth?	Crown above the gum. Enamel, dentine, pulp cavity and root canal. Root below the gum.
How many teeth are there in each quadrant?	Two incisors. One canine. Two premolars. Three molars (including the wisdom teeth).
What is the nerve and blood supply of the alveolar bones?	Superior alveolar nerve (maxillary CN V2). Inferior alveolar nerve (mandibular CN V3). Superior alveolar artery (maxillary). Inferior alveolar artery (maxillary).

Table 6.1 Eye muscles

Muscle	Origin	Course	Insertion	Action	Innervation
Superior rectus	Common tendinous ring (annulus of Zinn)	Fibres pass forwards around eyeball	Sclera on superior surface of eyeball	Elevates, adducts and medially rotates the eye	Oculomotor n. (superior br.)
Inferior rectus	Common tendinous ring (annulus of Zinn)	Fibres pass forwards around eyeball	Sclera on inferior surface of eyeball	Depresses, adducts and laterally rotates the eye	Oculomotor n. (inferior br.)
Medial rectus	Common tendinous ring (annulus of Zinn)	Fibres pass forwards around eyeball	Sclera on medial surface of eyeball	Adducts the eyeball	Oculomotor n. (inferior br.)
Lateral rectus	Common tendinous ring (annulus of Zinn)	Fibres pass forwards around eyeball	Sclera on lateral surface of eyeball	Abducts eye	Abducent n.
Superior oblique	Bone above tendinous ring	Fibres travel forwards along upper border of medial rectus, through the trochlea and then posteriorly	Sclera on posterior superior surface of eyeball	Intorsion, depresses and abducts eyeball	Trochlear n.
Inferior oblique	Floor of orbit, lateral to lacrimal groove	Fibres pass laterally, backwards and upwards between inferior rectus and floor of orbit	Sclera on inferior surface of eyeball	Extorsion, elevates and abduction	Oculomotor n.

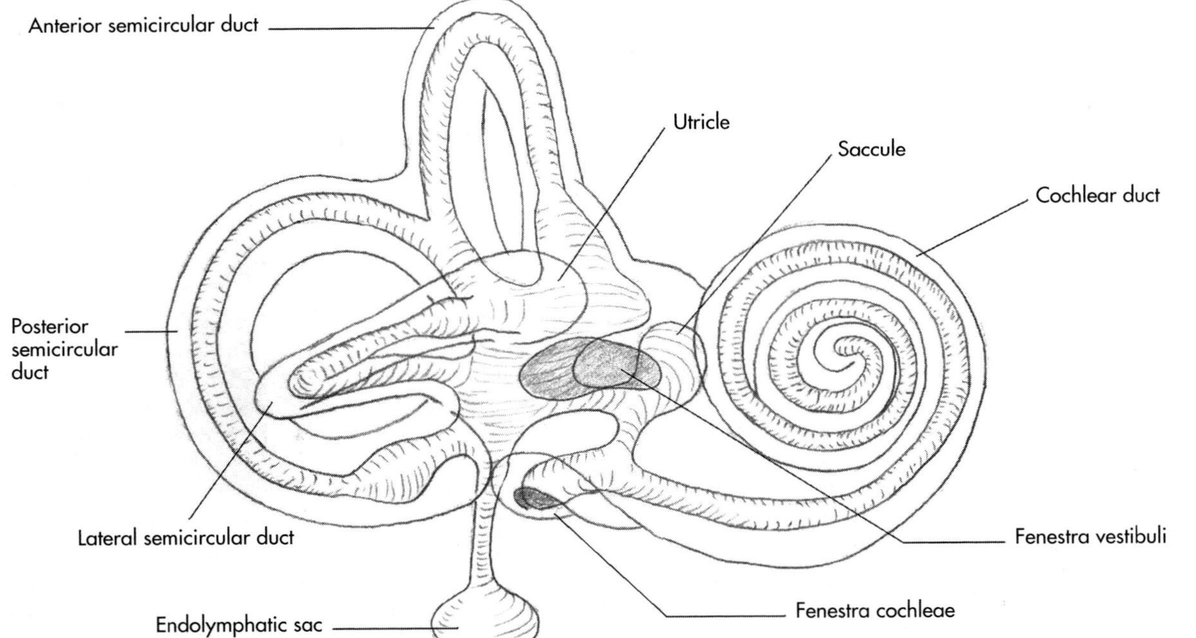

Figure 6.1 The inner ear showing the membranous labyrinth within the bony labyrinth

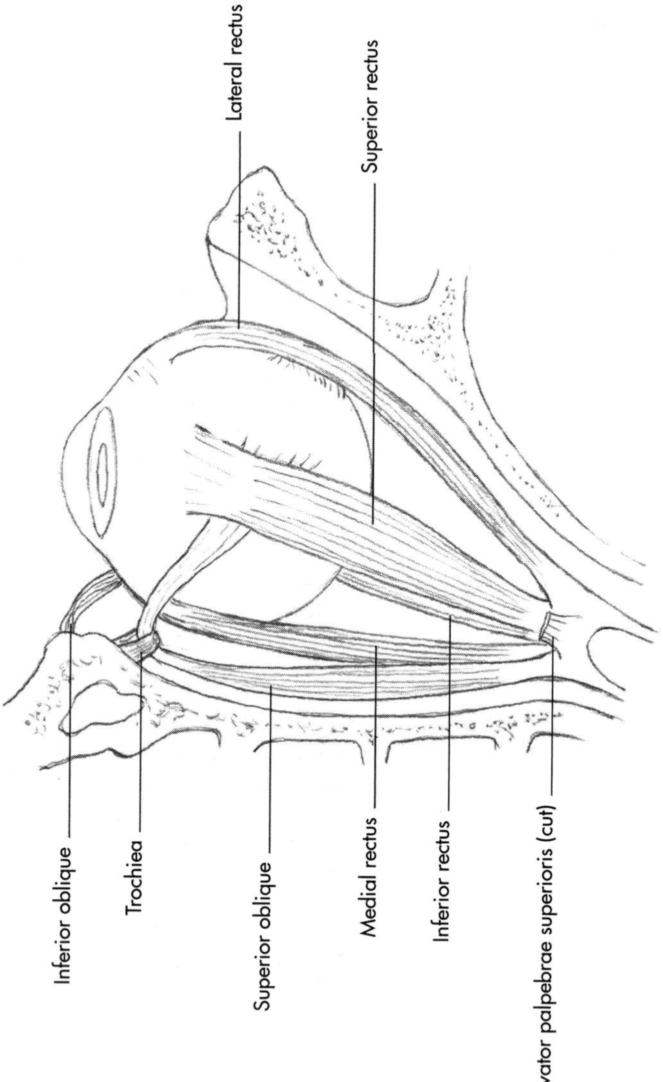

Figure 6.2 Extraocular muscles, superior view

CHAPTER 7: ENDOCRINE GLANDS

ADRENAL GLAND

What does the adrenal gland produce?

Depends on the area. It comprises an outer cortex and an inner medulla.
The cortex has three zones:
(*Mnemonic:* from outside in, **GFR** [remembered by the fact that the adrenal sits atop the kidney where the glomerular filtration rate, or GFR, is important!].)
1. **Zona Glomerulosa** (outer): mineralocorticoids.
2. **Zona Fasciculata** (middle): glucocorticoids and androgens.
3. **Zona Reticulata** (inner): oestrogens.

80% of cathecolamines produced by the adrenal medulla is in the form of epinephrine, and 10% is in the form of norepinepherine.

What is the main glucocorticoid?

Cortisol.

How is it controlled?

Via a feedback loop: **corticotrophin-releasing hormone** (**CRH**) from the anterior hypothalamus stimulates **adrenocorticotrophic hormone** (**ACTH**) release from the anterior pituitary, which in turn stimulates cortisol release from the adrenal gland. Cortisol negatively feeds back to CRH and ACTH.

What is the main mineralocorticoid?

Aldosterone.

How is it controlled?

The **renin–angiotensin–aldosterone axis.** A fall in blood pressure is sensed as renal perfusion by the kidney, which causes renin release from its juxtaglomerular apparatus. This stimulates angiotensin (and its active metabolite angiotensin II) production in the lung, which has a direct vasoconstrictive effect and causes aldosterone release from the adrenal gland. Aldosterone causes salt retention by acting on the collecting ducts of the kidney.

THYROID GLAND

What is the thyroid gland?

An endocrine gland (a ductless gland secreting hormones directly into bloodstream) with control over metabolic rate through thyroxine (T_4) and triiodothyronine (T_3), stimulated by thyroid-stimulating hormone (TSH) from the anterior pituitary gland.

Where does it lie?

The gland consists of two lobes communicating anteriorly by the 'isthmus'. It is this isthmus that lies on the anterior trachea at the second and third tracheal rings. The whole gland is attached to the pretracheal fascia.

What is a goitre?

An enlargement of the gland. There are three varieties of goitre:
1. Diffuse goitre.
2. Multinodular goitre.
3. Solitary nodule.

Goitres can extend to the superior mediastinum.

What is the blood supply to the thyroid gland?

Two superior thyroid arteries (from the external carotid) dividing into anterior and posterior branches. Two inferior thyroid arteries (from thyrocervical trunk, subclavian)

passing behind the gland. It has a close relation to the recurrent laryngeal nerve.
A thyroidea ima artery occasionally appears directly from the brachiocephalic trunk inferiorly.

What is the venous drainage?

Superior and middle veins drain to the internal jugular. The inferior drains to the brachiocephalic.

What two nerves must be preserved during thyroidectomy?

The recurrent laryngeal and superior laryngeal nerves.

Where does the recurrent laryngeal nerve run?

Lateral to the gland on both sides, in the tracheo-oesophageal groove.

What is its relationship to the inferior thyroid artery?

Usually behind the artery on the left, but has a 50% chance of being either in front of or behind the artery on the right.

How are these two nerves preserved during thyroidectomy?

By clamping the superior thyroid artery *at* the superior thyroid pole (where it enters), hence preserving the superior laryngeal nerve, and by clamping the inferior thyroid artery *lateral* to the inferior pole (where it enters), hence preserving the recurrent laryngeal nerve.

What is the thyroglossal tract?

It is a remnant of the thyroglossal duct in which the thyroid gland develops and descends from the foramen caecum of the tongue. An incomplete regression results in a cyst found within the tract. Protrusion of the tongue will cause the cyst to rise as a result of the tract's attachment to the tongue.

PARATHYROID GLANDS

Where are the parathyroid glands?

Usually behind the superior and inferior poles of the thyroid gland. The position of the two superior glands is more constant, whereas the inferior glands can be quite variable in position (e.g. in thyroid substance, lower neck or mediastinum). There are four in all.

What is the function of the parathyroid glands?

They secrete parathyroid hormone (PTH) and calcitonin, which are involved with calcium homeostasis.

From where do the parathyroids originate?

Superior glands: fourth pharyngeal pouch.
Inferior glands: third pharyngeal pouch (same as the thymus, which displaces them caudally, accounting for their sometimes variable positions).

How is serum calcium regulated?

See Figure 7.1.

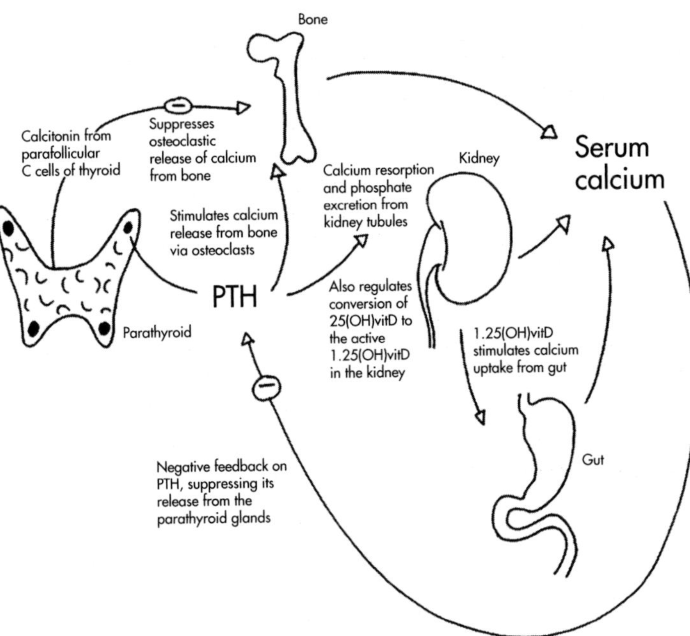
Bone
Calcitonin from parafollicular C cells of thyroid
Suppresses osteoclastic release of calcium from bone
Serum calcium
Kidney
Calcium resorption and phosphate excretion from kidney tubules
Stimulates calcium release from bone via osteoclasts
PTH
Parathyroid
Also regulates conversion of 25(OH)vitD to the active 1.25(OH)vitD in the kidney
1.25(OH)vitD stimulates calcium uptake from gut
Gut
Negative feedback on PTH, suppressing its release from the parathyroid glands

Figure 7.1

INDEX

a, note about adjectives: right/left greater/lesser deep/superficial inferior/superior common, middle, lateral, medial oblique, ant/pst not alpabetized